D1557676

THE UNDESCENDED TESTIS

The Undescended Testis

ERIC W. FONKALSRUD, M.D.

Professor and Chief, Pediatric Surgery
University of California, Los Angeles
School of Medicine
Los Angeles, California

WOLFGANG MENGEL, M.D.

Department for General Surgery
Christian-Albrechts-University of Kiel
Kiel, West Germany

YEAR BOOK MEDICAL PUBLISHERS, INC.
CHICAGO • LONDON

Copyright © 1981 by Year Book Medical Publishers, Inc. All rights reserved. No part of this publication may be reproduced, stored in a retrieval system, or transmitted, in any form or by any means, electronic, mechanical, photocopying, recording, or otherwise, without prior written permission from the publisher. Printed in the United States of America.

Library of Congress Cataloging in Publication Data
Main entry under title:

The undescended testis.

    Includes index.
    1. Cryptorchidism.   I. Fonkalsrud, E. W.
II. Mengel, Wolfgang. [DNLM: 1. Cryptorchidism.
WJ840 U56]
RJ477.5.C74U52   618.92'68   80-19479
ISBN 0-8151-3257-3

To the children of today and tomorrow, from the children of yesterday and from the contributing authors, who have shared their special expertise to provide better care for the young of the future

Foreword

Orchiopexy is the third most common major surgical operation performed by children's surgeons. Two hundred and thirty recently certified pediatric surgeons reported that 5% of some 75,000 operations involved the correction of this poorly understood congenital malformation, which occurs in nearly 1% of the male population. Thus, Fonkalsrud and Mengel's book deals with a surprisingly common problem. Because of the international representation of the authors, this timely volume should provide more standardization in the management of individual children who are born with the "empty scrotum" syndrome. When 22 authors from 12 institutions in 6 different countries converge on the cryptorchid male, the results should be rewarding—and this volume is!

From the Introduction to the concluding Summary, authoritative discussions are presented on the embryogenesis of the malformation, problems in its diagnosis, potential adverse effects, and the methods and results of a wide variety of therapies in different age groups. Although this multiauthored approach leads to obvious overlapping of information and duplication in the bibliography, the repetition, particularly of significant new data, proves to be highly desirable.

The volume reviews the most current available information on the *untreated* cryptorchid infant with unilateral or bilateral disease. Associated endocrinopathies, potential for spontaneous descent, expectation for endocrine function as well as reproductive potential, and the threat of subsequent malignant degeneration are all dealt with. Well documented is the relative effectiveness of exogenous HCG and LH-RH. A variety of well-described surgical procedures for increasingly younger patients is encouraged.

In short, the *selection of timing* for treatment need no longer depend on a few facts, fallacies, and the size of the cord structures. This book stands as a biomedical anatomical resource, emphasizing a "reasonable" approach to individual patients.

What is unique about this book is that it presents to the pediatrician and generalist a single source of the most up-to-date information on cryptorchidism—a guide for decision making on a matter of great importance to infant patients and their families. For physicians and surgeons, the specifics of recommended treatments and anticipated results are fully discussed and well illustrated.

The authors conclude that patients with impalpable or bilaterally undescended testes or with other major congénital syndromes are individuals who need a "team approach." However, the child with unilateral ectopia or presumably "mechanical" nondescent so often associated with a hernia needs a single surgical procedure, usually during the second year of life. If consideration for treatment has been delayed until the mid or late teens, testicular biopsy to identify dysplastic testes and occult carcinoma is mandatory. In unilateral cases, orchidectomy may be the most conservative approach.

These generalizations are well supported on the basis of anatomical, histologic, and more recent functional follow-up studies. Since the past treatment programs have left much to be desired, the factual information provided in this volume should improve the understanding and management of the cryptorchid male and will undoubtedly encourage further studies and discourse.

H. WILLIAM CLATWORTHY, JR., M.D.

Department of Pediatric Surgery
Columbus Children's Hospital
Columbus, Ohio

Preface

Cryptorchidism is one of the most common malformations encountered in males, yet there is greater controversy regarding the pathophysiology of the condition and the optimal form of treatment than for almost any other anomaly currently amenable to medical and/or surgical management. A vast amount of information on the subject is available in isolated reports and reviews, often providing somewhat controversial and inconclusive data. Thus it is difficult for the practicing physician to clearly determine which course of treatment is optimal for specific patients with undescended testes.

After a monograph on the subject "The Undescended Testis" was published in *Current Problems in Surgery* in 1978, it became readily apparent that many of the controversial aspects of the malformation should be expanded by authorities in the field and compiled into one volume. Despite the many variable approaches still recommended for the management of cryptorchidism, no other comprehensive volume on the condition has been published during the past decade.

The aim of this book is to provide a foundation of information regarding most aspects of cryptorchidism. Not all of the contributing authors concur on how best to manage children with the anomaly. By presenting information and data supporting the different points of view, it is hoped the reader will become sufficiently well informed to make his own judgment.

Eric W. Fonkalsrud

Wolfgang Mengel

Contributors

BACKHOUSE, KENNETH M., O.B.E., V.R.D.
Professor, Department of Anatomy, Charing Cross Hospital Medical School, The Royal College of Surgeons of England, London

BERCU, BARRY B., M.D.
Division of Pediatric Surgery, Massachusetts General Hospital, Boston, Massachusetts; National Institutes of Health, Bethesda, Maryland

CYWES, SYDNEY, M. MED. (SURG.), F.A.C.S.
Professor and Head, Department of Pediatric Surgery, University of Cape Town; Red Cross War Memorial Children's Hospital, Cape Town, South Africa

DONAHOE, PATRICIA K., M.D.
Associate Professor, Division of Surgery, Harvard Medical School; Massachusetts General Hospital, Boston

FONKALSRUD, ERIC W., M.D.
Professor and Chief of Pediatric Surgery, University of California, Los Angeles, School of Medicine

GEFFNER, MITCHELL E., M.D.
Fellow, Department of Pediatrics, Division of Pediatric Endocrinology and Metabolism, University of California, Los Angeles, School of Medicine

GINSBURG, HOWARD B., M.D.
Division of Pediatric Surgery, Harvard Medical School; Massachusetts General Hospital, Boston

GIRARD, J., M.D.
Basel Children's Hospital, Basel, Switzerland

GROSFELD, JAY L., M.D.
Professor and Chief of Pediatric Surgery, Indiana University School of Medicine; Surgeon-in-Chief, James Whitcomb Riley Hospital for Children, Indianapolis, Indiana

HADŽISELIMOVIC, FARUK, Ph.D.
Basel Children's Hospital, Basel, Switzerland

HECKER, W. CH., M.D.
Professor and Chief, Clinic of Pediatric Surgery, University Children's Hospital, Munich, West Germany

HENDREN, W. HARDY, M.D.
Professor and Chief, Division of Pediatric Surgery, Harvard Medical School; Massachusetts General Hospital, Boston

HINMAN, FRANK, JR., M.D.
Professor and Chief, Department of Urology, University of California, San Francisco, School of Medicine

KNORR, D., M.D.
Professor, Department of Pediatrics and Chief of Endocrinology, University Children's Hospital, Munich, West Germany

LIPPE, BARBARA M., M.D.
Associate Professor, Department of Pediatrics, Division of Pediatric Endocrinology and Metabolism, University of California, Los Angeles, School of Medicine

LOUW, JAN H., M.CH., F.R.C.S., F.A.C.S.
Professor and Head, Department of Surgery, University of Cape Town; Red Cross War Memorial Children's Hospital, Cape Town, South Africa

MARTIN, DONALD C., M.D.
Professor and Chief, Division of Urology, University of California, Irvine, College of Medicine

MENGEL, WOLFGANG, M.D.
Department for General Surgery, Christian-Albrechts-University of Kiel, Kiel, West Germany

RADHAKRISHNAN, JAYANT, M.D.
Chief, Division of Pediatric Surgery, Cook County Hospital, Chicago

RETIEF, P.J.M., M.B., CH.B., CH.M.
Consultant Urologist, Department of Pediatric Surgery, Red Cross War Memorial Children's Hospital, Cape Town, South Africa

WRONECKI, KRYSTOF, M.D.
Pediatric Surgery Unit, University Hospital, Wroclaw, Poland

ZIMMERMANN, FRANZ A., M.D.
Clinic of Pediatric Surgery, University Children's Hospital, Munich, West Germany

Contents

1 / Introduction

ERIC W. FONKALSRUD, M.D.

ONE OF THE EARLIEST recorded accounts of undescended testes is thought to have been written in 1786 by John Hunter,[1] who observed that the testis is located in the abdomen until the seventh month of fetal development and by the ninth month has moved into the scrotum in most normal male infants. He believed that the descent of the testis was directed by a cord or ligament, which he termed the "gubernaculum," although he surmised that the fault of maldescent originated in the testes themselves. He further noted that "when one or both testes remain throughout life in the belly, they are exceedingly imperfect and probably incapable of performing their natural function." Hunter also stated that if the testis has been arrested in its descent in infancy, "I think the completion most frequently happens between the years of two and ten." Although considerable information has been acquired regarding the embryologic development of the testes, the hormonal influences affecting descent, the morphologic features of the undescended compared to the normally descended testis, the function of the undescended testes, and many other pathophysiologic aspects of the anomaly during the 200 years since Hunter's original observations, many of his concepts are still valid.

The word "cryptorchid" comes from the Greek words *cryptos*, meaning hidden, and *orchis*, meaning testis, and thus literally is "hidden testis." This term is frequently applied to all forms of undescended testes, both palpable and nonpalpable, and generally refers to the presence of an empty scrotum. The word "cryptorchidism" is almost interchangeable with the term "undescended testis" except that the latter does not include gonads that may be manipulated into the scrotum, e.g., "retractile testes." The reason for incomplete descent remains somewhat unclear but a thorough knowledge of the embryologic development, as well as an understanding of the hormonal influences on descent and development of the gonad, is essential in planning a rational approach to treatment.

Prior to 1900 a patient with an undescended testis usually was advised to ignore the condition. In those rare circumstances when the patient underwent operation, the undescended testis generally was removed.[2] By 1899 a definite change in the management of the undescended testis was developed when Bevan[2] suggested that orchiopexy should be considered for some adults with testicular undescent. Four years later he expressed confidence in surgical repair for cryptorchidism and recommended operation for most patients during the early teen-age years rather than in adult life.[3] The operative repair, placing the cryptorchid testes into the scrotum, has been refined during the past 75 years, and today it is performed with low risk and high success by most pediatric surgeons. Various operative techniques have been developed to place even the high intra-abdominal testes into the scrotum. Moreover, even testicular transplantation using microsurgical techniques has been performed in certain clinical situations.

There are two main viewpoints regarding the cause of the undescended testis: (1) it is an inherently "sick" testis lacking the capacity for normal development, and its failure to descend into the scrotum reflects this abnormality; and (2) it is a potentially normal testis, hampered in its development by its unfriendly environment, and a satisfactory orchiopexy at the optimal time will restore it to normal function. The implications of the first viewpoint are that orchiopexy neither improves spermatogenesis nor prevents the complications of nondescent, including malignancy. Indications for the operation are therefore limited to the desire to correct an associated clinical hernia or to prevent psychologic disturbances resulting from an empty, undeveloped scrotum. In the absence of these relatively rare complications, clinical observation without treatment might be recommended or orchiectomy might be performed as cancer prophylaxis. On the other hand, those who accept the second viewpoint recommend orchiopexy with or without prior gonadotropin administration. Advocates of this concept have attempted to design operative techniques that will permit proper placement of the testis into the scrotum without injury to its blood supply and function. During the past few decades, there has been a gradual shift of opinion toward the second approach.

Formerly the results of orchiopexy were judged by the postoperative position and size of the testes. Only in the case of bilateral cryptorchidism could subsequent paternity or semen examination be used as an index of the benefit of the operation. The more widespread use of testicular biopsy in the past two decades has provided a direct, objective method of determining the changes caused by orchiopexy. By serial testicular biopsies during and following operation, an accu-

rate kinetic view can now be obtained showing progressive morphological changes in the seminiferous tubules and developing spermatogonia. It is no longer necessary to wait until a child reaches adulthood
to evaluate the results of operation, since biopsies will accurately indicate the degree of improvement in tubular structure and spermatogenesis resulting from scrotal positioning of the gonad. Furthermore,
comparative histologic study of the undescended and of the scrotal
testis at various ages has disclosed more precisely the time at which
deleterious effects of cryptorchidism begin. Nonetheless, semen analysis and sperm counts provide the most accurate indication of the
effectiveness of orchiopexy in increasing the incidence of fertility.

During the past three quarters of a century since Bevan's original
recommendation for orchiopexy, surgical therapy for undescended
testes has gained wide acceptance, and there has been a gradual
lowering of the recommended age for operative repair. Many patients
have had no improvement in histologic appearance of the gonad or
spermatogenic function when the repair has been performed after
normal growth is underway or has been completed, thus suggesting
that orchiopexy be performed before the onset of puberty. Many physicians now believe that the undescended testis that remains elevated
in the pubescent male should be treated by orchiectomy rather than
by orchiopexy. Certain contraindications for orchiopexy have been
described under specific circumstances, although agreement on this
issue is not unanimous. Human chorionic gonadotropin (HCG) therapy has frequently been provided for boys with testicular undescent,
although the indications for its use and the results following treatment
have varied widely in different clinics.

Although a statistically significant correlation exists between undescended testes and the development of testicular malignancy, the exact
relationship is not clearly defined. It appears that the more hypoplastic the gonad the greater the likelihood of subsequent malignant
change. The therapeutic success of orchiopexy or hormone therapy in
preventing malignant change or in achieving normal spermatogenesis
has been the subject of considerable speculation and controversy.
Despite these unsettled issues, the currently recommended rational
therapy for managing cryptorchid testes rests on an extensive background of clinical observation and basic investigation.

The undescended testis is one of the most common anomalies encountered in males, and yet there is greater controversy regarding the
pathophysiologic nature of the condition and the optimal form of treatment than for almost any other malformation currently amenable to
surgical reconstruction. Furthermore, there is a large volume of infor-

mation available in isolated reports and reviews on the subject, which provides somewhat controversial and inconclusive data, thus making it difficult for the practicing physician to determine clearly which course of therapy is optimal for specific patients. The purpose of this volume, therefore, is to provide a consensus regarding the practical aspects of managing the undescended testes as compiled by several authorities in the field.

REFERENCES

1. Hunter J.: in Palmer R. (ed.): *Observations on Certain Parts of the Animal Economy*. London, Longmans, Green & Co., 1785.
2. Bevan A.D.: Operation for undescended testicle and congenital inguinal hernia. *J.A.M.A.* 33:773, 1899.
3. Bevan A.D.: The surgical treatment of undescended testicle. *J.A.M.A.* 41:718, 1903.

2 / Embryology of the Normal and Cryptorchid Testis

KENNETH M. BACKHOUSE, O.B.E., V.R.D.

THE TESTIS IN VERTEBRATE animals develops on the posterior abdominal wall in relation to the mesonephros, the temporary segmental
kidney of the embryonic period, and its duct. It then takes over part of
the mesonephric duct system once the metanephric system has developed and in most animals, including many mammals, remains
more or less in situ. For some reason the human testis, as well as that
of most other mammals, has evolved a mechanism for escaping from
the abdomen to a vulnerable site outside. Why this should have taken
place is obscure, unless it is a manifestation of the sexual exhibition
that is so frequent, varied, and often bizarre in biologic systems. Whatever the reason, in so doing it has resulted in the evolution of a biochemical system, particularly for spermatogenic activity, with a narrow optimal temperature range markedly lower than that of the abdomen and also of the testes of those animals that retain them in the abdomen. To argue, as many do, that the testes must descend into the
scrotum to achieve a cool environment seems untenable since, even
among mammals (elephant, hyrax, and all whales and dolphins), as
well as birds, the testes function effectively at the higher intra-abdominal temperature. Although seals, like all carnivores, show testicular descent, they differ in that the testes descend very early in fetal
life but are retained at the external inguinal ring deep to the thick fat
and remain there at body temperature. In man and other mammals
with extra-abdominal testes and hence a low temperature system, disorders of developmental gonad location can have a disastrous effect,
particularly on spermatogenic function.

For this reason, many mammals, including man, have a tempera-
ture-controlled dartos muscle in the scrotal wall, which, acting with
the countercurrent temperature effect of the testicular artery and its
closely applied pampiniform plexus, maintains a fairly even tempera-

5

ture. In addition, the cremaster muscle is available as a testicle retracting defense mechanism, but this becomes far less active as a retractile element once the testis is fully secreting its hormones in active sexual life.

NORMAL TESTICULAR DEVELOPMENT

Human gonads develop on the posterior abdominal wall just caudal to the developing suprarenal cortex in the region between the dorsal mesentery and the mesonephros, i.e., a ridge of tissue eventually destined to produce steroids. At about four weeks (4–5 mm crown-rump [C-R] length), a proliferation of the coelomic epithelium and a thickening of the underlying mesenchyma encroach onto the medial aspect of the developing mesonephric ridge. The epithelial cells in this coelomic ridge remain cuboid to columnar, whereas the remainder of the epithelium differentiates to a more mature pavement-like appearance; these cells also remain without the basement membrane that develops elsewhere. The absence of this basement membrane allows the proliferating epithelial cells to penetrate into the underlying mesenchyma. These cells in their proliferation form irregular cordlike arrangements, initially connected with the surface epithelium, and are known as the primitive sex cords. Thus as the gonadal swelling progresses, much of its bulk is formed by this epithelial invasion.

Meanwhile the primordial germ cells or gonocytes have been forming and moving into the region. These are larger, more rounded cells with large vesicular nuclei and considerable cytoplasm, which stains less well than that of the other gonadic cells. Such cells appear much earlier and are now generally recognized to have originated in the wall of the yolk sac close to the allantois, whence they have migrated along the mesentery to the gonad.[1]

It has been suggested that the arrival of the primordial germ cells actively induces the changes in the gonadic ridge, but in man they do not become evident in the area until about the sixth week, by which time the ridges are prominent. On their arrival, the primordial germ cells come to lie both in the epithelium and in the superficial layers of the underlying mesenchyma. As the sex cords form from the epithelium, the germ cells become contained within the cords and carried with them into the underlying mesenchyma. Thus the as yet undifferentiated gonad consists of cells from three sources: primordial germ cell, coelomic epithelial sex cords, and mesenchymal stroma into which the first two have migrated.

By the end of the sixth week of the embryonic period, the testis begins to differ from the ovary. During the next two weeks (15–25 mm C-R length), the sex cords continue to proliferate into the medulla and, with their contained primordial germ cells, become well formed into a branching system. The connections of the cords with the surface epithelium is lost, and by the time the 25-mm length is reached, there is evidence of the differentiation of fibroblasts that will form the tunica albuginea; thereafter the coelomic epithelium remains only as the peritoneal cover.

In the deepest part of the structure, the cords break up into a finer network of strand cells, which eventually form the rete testis in the region of the mesorchium. With later development the cords become canalized, their walls containing the germ cells and the fetal sustentacular (Sertoli) cells. The rete testis, on the other hand, becomes canalized later still (between 50 mm and 90 mm C-R length) and, by extension into the tissue of the mesonephric ridge, links up with a number of the mesonephric tubules. This gives the seminiferous tubules their linkage via the efferent ductules with the mesonephric duct.

The mesenchymatous tissue between the cords differentiates into fibroblasts and into Leydig (interstitial) cells, which become active early in fetal life. Giroud[2] considered them to be most active during the three to five months of intrauterine life. Jost[3] produced incontrovertible evidence of hormonal activity in development, and thereafter studies were made attempting to elucidate when and where fetal testosterone was produced. It rapidly became evident that a fetal mammalian testis was capable of producing steroid hormones (at least in vitro) before the interstitial cells were recognizable (by use of the light microscope). In man, 3-hydroxysteroid dehydrogenase, an enzyme essential to testosterone production, is demonstrable in the mesenchyma of the gonadic ridge before it can be shown in interstitial cells, according to Baillie et al.[4] However, in other mammals, Black and Christensen[5] noted smooth endoplasmic reticulum, known to be associated with the production of steroid hormones, in the mesenchyma cells in their early development. In man, by using ultrastructural evidence, Holstein et al.[6] considered that mesenchyma cells could be shown to differentiate into Leydig cells by eight weeks, with marked increase in their size and activity between the ninth and 12th weeks, reaching a maximum during the 17th week of pregnancy. Thus even in the early stages of development, steroid hormones and probably testosterone are produced before the testis is fully recognized histologically; later they can be shown to be produced principally by the interstitial cells, but some also by the fetal Sertoli cells. Male hormones are thus available at the time of embryonic differentiation from the neutral (largely female) form to the male, with the necessary changes in duct form and development of male structure.

DEVELOPMENT OF THE GUBERNACULUM TESTIS AND DUCT SYSTEM

The testis, being formed in relation to the mesonephric duct, becomes secondarily connected with it through the rete testis. The paramesonephric duct also is related and this runs with the mesonephric duct in the mesonephric ridge to the pelvis. In the embryo, development of the pelvic region is tardy, and the prominent mesonephric ridge or fold (and initially even the mesonephros) fills a major part of the existing lateral pelvic space so that the fold lies virtually in contact with the future inguinal region. In this way a link is readily established between the mesonephric ridge and the future inguinal region, which becomes identifiable as the inguinal ridge or fold once the pelvic cavity becomes more developed. Thus a mesenchymatous ridge now runs from the gonad and the mesonephros to the anterior abdominal wall in the inguinal region, the upper part containing the mesonephric and paramesonephric ducts, until they turn toward the midline; the lower part, the inguinal fold, crosses the umbilical artery. This fold from gonad to inguinal region may be called the plica gubernaculi or intra-abdominal gubernaculum.

The genital swellings meanwhile are forming, and in the mesenchyma of the body wall the muscles are differentiating. The muscles actually can be seen early in the sixth week (10 – 12 mm). However, in the inguinal region a deficiency occurs in the formation of the body wall musculature (Fig 2 – 1) that is similar in form to the gaps in muscular development occurring around the nerves, but far more extensive; in fact, the genital branch of the genitofemoral nerve runs through this muscular gap, as may the ilio-inguinal nerve (although this usually has a separate opening through the external oblique muscle). There is thus a mesenchyma-filled deficiency in the developing abdominal muscles at the inguinal canal, i.e., a preformed opening or canal in the body wall muscle. This is the future inguinal canal. A column of mesenchyma runs from the developing testis as a peritoneal covered fold in the abdomen to the inguinal canal and then through this into the future scrotal (or labial) swelling (Fig 2 – 2). This mesenchymatous column is the gubernaculum, and it is important to appreciate its totally undifferentiated mesenchymatous nature; its intra-abdominal part[7, 8] does of course contain the ducts.

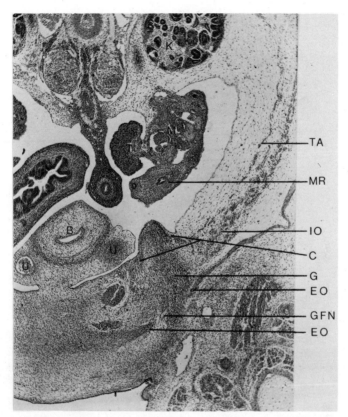

Fig 2–1. – Section through caudal part of 23-mm C-R length human embryo including future inguinal region. *T* = testis; *M* = mesonephros; *MR* = mesonephric ridge; *K* = metonephric kidney; *B* = bladder; *U* = umbilical arteries; *TA* = transversus abdominis muscle; *IO* = internal oblique muscle; *EO* = external oblique showing the two edges at external inguinal ring; *GFN* = genitofemoral nerve passing out of external inguinal ring, *G* = gubernaculum; *C* = early differentiation of cremaster muscle apparently running to inguinal fold, which can be seen bulging into abdominal cavity. Condensation of gubernacular mesenchyma may be seen running from fold out through gap in external oblique aponeurosis toward genital region.

With sexual differentiation (and this appears to accompany the initiation of steroid production by the mesenchymal cells differentiating to interstitial cells of the testis), the paramesonephric duct degenerates in the male, leaving only the mesonephric duct to become, in part, the vas deferens. The external genital swellings also take on male form.

Prior to sexual differentiation, two changes have occurred in the

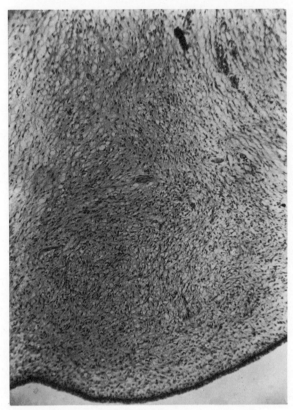

Fig 2–2.—Gubernacular mesenchyma in scrotal region of 45-mm C-R length human embryo.

mesenchyma in the inguinal region. Some time after the anterior abdominal wall muscles are laid down (late in the seventh week at about the 22- to 23-mm stage), new muscle cells differentiate into the cremaster muscle, which develops in the region of the future cremasteric origins from the inguinal ligament (lateral cremaster) and the pubis (medial cremaster), extending into the periphery of the gubernacular mesenchyma within the inguinal region. Initially the muscle fibers appear to grow into the gubernacular fold toward the testis (see Fig 2–1), but this is only transient and, as the body wall thickens, may become limited to the inguinal canal region. There is no question of an inverted cremaster muscle running up to the abdominal testis as ascribed to Hunter[9] and repeated in many descriptions. In fact, Hunter states that, if in a fetus the intra-abdominal testis is pulled upward, the cremaster fibers can be seen in the gubernaculum; presumably he pulled them up from the inguinal region.

While the cremaster muscle is developing, a gutter forms around the junction of the intra-abdominal gubernacular fold with the abdominal wall. This is the beginning of the processus vaginalis. It is difficult at this stage to be certain whether this small processus develops by active coelomic (peritoneal) epithelial invasion into the gubernacular mesenchyma of the inguinal region or whether the effect is produced by thickening of the surrounding body wall. At this stage the processus is very small relative to the body wall thickness and remains so for a considerable time after its formation. It has not been possible to show an increase in coelomic epithelial cell division that would indicate active invasion as the processus vaginalis forms, although this occurs later around the time of testicular descent when there is more rapid growth of the processus. Whatever the actual mechanism, there is a small beginning of the processus vaginalis into the gubernacular mesenchyma in the inguinal canal and, once this has formed effectively, the cremaster muscle remains peripheral to the processus vaginalis. It does not grow into the extension of the intra-abdominal gubernacular fold separated within the inguinal canal by the processus vaginalis.

Thus the cremaster muscles and the processus vaginalis can be seen to develop in the gubernacular mesenchyma of the inguinal region in rudimentary form in both sexes before effective sexual differentiation; they will progress later in the male but not in the female.

The male is now prepared for future developments and eventual testicular descent. The testis and the mesonephros, over which it originally partially lay, have been connected with the posterior body wall and the diaphragm, but as the mesonephros degenerates, these cranial connections are lost, leaving the testis free at its upper pole. Its lower pole is connected by its mesenchymatous gubernacular fold to the inguinal region and through this by undifferentiated mesenchyma into the core of the scrotal swelling (see Fig 2–2). The cremaster muscle differentiates in the inguinal region of the gubernacular mesenchyma within which it can later extend distally by further differentiation. The processus vaginalis is likewise initiated and will later extend distally by active coelomic epithelial invasion into the gubernacular mesenchyma separating from a central extension of the abdominal gubernacular mesenchyma fold. However, for the moment the more distal gubernacular mesenchyma remains, filling the inguinal canal and future scrotum, a mesenchymatous residuum as the body wall structures differentiate and develop.

At this stage in man, a period of quiescence ensues once the male reproductive components have begun to develop. The fetal body wall will continue to grow, in particular the pelvic region, which is slower to develop than the initially more vital cranial structures. As the body grows, so the testis, on its mesentery with its gubernaculum column linked to the inguinal region, gradually becomes more caudal, i.e., there is a relative descent as the lumbar and pelvic regions develop.

With growth of the body wall, its undifferentiated mesenchyma between, inside, and outside the abdominal muscles gradually becomes converted to fasciae. The most obvious changes can be seen from about 100 mm (16 weeks) onward, with gradual formation of the membranous components of the superficial fascia. This differentiation extends to the mesenchyma at the future external inguinal ring and thence forms a layer beneath the scrotal skin. Just as the muscles did not form in the mesenchyma of the gubernaculum at the inguinal region, so the developing fascia does not encroach here either (Figs 2–3 and 2–4). The distal end of the gubernacular mesenchyma now is contained in a differentiated pocket of the scrotal wall but still remains continuous through the inguinal canal with the testis above. The gubernaculum is still essentially undifferentiated mesenchyma, and the cremaster muscle and processus vaginalis are rudimentary (Fig 2–5).

It is perhaps convenient at this stage in human development, while there appears to be relative inactivity in the gubernaculum testis, to consider what happens in certain other animals that proceed similarly to testicular descent and have been used by various authors either for experimental studies or by descriptive inference to explain the mechanisms of testicular descent in man. However, there is a wide species variation in the process that makes interspecific extrapolation difficult and often grossly misleading. This fact, together with frank misquoting of references, particularly those of Hunter, has created many problems in the past; for instance, Seiler,[10] and also many others, reported that Hunter had shown that an ascending cremaster muscle pulled the testis into the scrotum. On the contrary, Hunter had actually claimed this to be impossible. Seiler than followed his misquotation of Hunter by stating that in adult sexual activity the testes of certain rodents (rat, squirrel) are taken into the abdomen and pulled out again into the scrotum by the cremaster; no feature of this description in the rat or squirrel on our evidence is correct.[11]

Another piece of incredible though generally accepted evidence was produced by Cloquet[12] and later by Carus,[13] who believed that loops of the abdominal muscles, particularly the internal oblique,

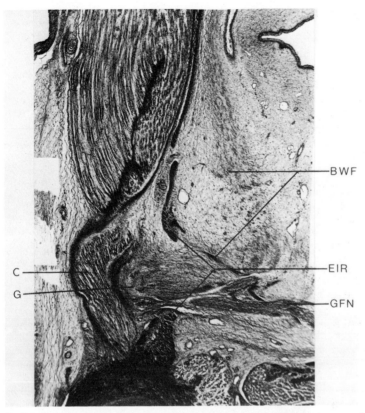

Fig 2–3.—Section through external inguinal ring of 127-mm human fetus, with body wall muscles to left and the superficial fascia to right. *EIR* = external inguinal ring in external oblique aponeurosis (note similar small aperture for nerve above); *C* = conjoint muscle (conjoint tendon in the adult); *G* = gubernaculum; *GFN* = genitofemoral nerve; *BWF* = beginning of differentiation of external body wall fascia, which may be seen forming condensation around gubernacular mesenchyma outside inguinal ring and extending to scrotal wall.

could frequently be found around an inguinal sac. Thus, they argued, as the gubernaculum develops, it herniates through the abdominal wall, carrying the various layers with it, which eventually cover the testis and cord. To adapt to this thesis, the cremaster muscle was described as being in loops separated from the lower margin of the internal oblique muscle. This looped cremaster muscle is still described in many textbooks of anatomy (Hollingshead,[14] Cunningham,[15] Gray,[16]), as is the development from the internal oblique muscle. Lemeh[17] repeats these views in a recent communication but presents no evi-

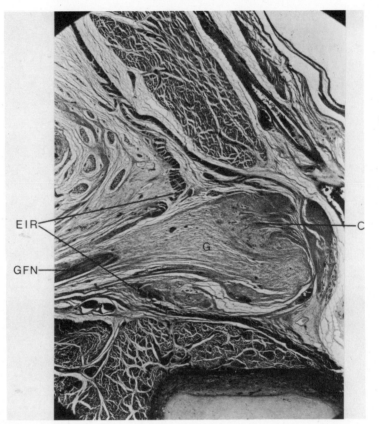

Fig 2–4.—Section through external inguinal ring (*EIR*) of 163-mm human fetus, with superficial fascia to left and body wall muscles and peritoneal cavity to right. *G* = gubernaculum passing through inguinal ring; *C* = cremaster muscle in inguinal canal; *GFN* = genitofemoral nerve. Note that superficial fascia is now well developed, as is fibrous tissue around gubernaculum outside ring.

dence in their support. Moreover, he claims that "during the descent of the testis, the abdominal musculature evaginates"—a statement that is inconsistent with the rest of his thesis.

As shown in Figures 2–1 and 2–3, the gubernaculum does not herniate through the abdominal wall but remains a mesenchymatous residuum as the abdominal wall structures develop around it in the inguinal canal and later in the scrotum. Thus the coverings of the future testis and cord do not fit in with the layers of the abdominal wall, nor is the cremaster looped to fit into a herniated internal oblique muscle.

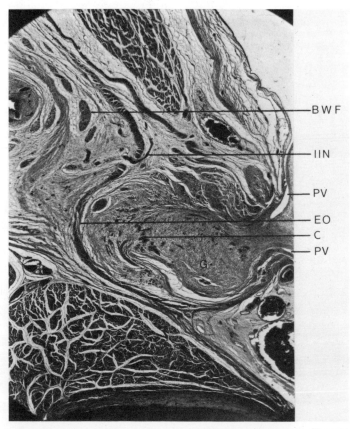

—BWF

—IIN

— PV

— EO
— C
— PV

Fig 2–5.—Similar section from same 163-mm fetus as in Figure 2–4 at internal ring and inguinal canal. *EO* = external oblique aponeurosis; *BWF* = superficial body wall fascia; *IIN* = ilio-inguinal nerve; *PV* = processus vaginalis; *C* = cremaster.

Even the supporters of the loop theory of cremasteric anatomy describe the medial cremaster portion of the loop as often absent. As we have shown, the cremaster muscle differentiates in the embryo at some time after differentiation of the body wall muscles and then only in fairly rudimentary form. It has a different nerve supply from the abdominal wall muscles, via the genitofemoral nerve to the genital region, which follows an entirely different course from the segmental body wall nerves. In postnatal life no interrelation exists between the internal oblique muscle and the cremaster either in electromyographic nerve or muscle stimulation studies, nor are there links between the muscles in local myopathic lesions. The cremaster muscle also can be shown to hypertrophy in certain circumstances under the influence of testosterone and to reduce its neuromuscular excitability in a way quite different from that of the internal oblique muscle.[18]

These developments may be said to occur in a comparable form in most mammals that have extra-abdominal testes but in which the later development and behavior of the testes vary so widely that no more than careful interspecific inferences can be made.

In rodents the process is considerably more continuous than in man; there is testicular descent by the time of birth into a bilaminar cremasteric sac as an abdominal extension. However, until puberty, the testis largely remains in the abdominal cavity, and the small cremasteric sac contains little more than the cauda epididymis. The course in insectivores follows a comparable pattern, with slightly more than the tail of the epididymis in the cremasteric sac. The ungulates that we examined and the pig, on which our original observations were made,[7] have a longer gestation, and their early development resembles that seen in man but then proceeds gradually to establish descent later in fetal life. For this reason they were valuable in demonstrating what happens far more rapidly in man. In certain carnivores, especially seals, testicular descent occurs remarkably early in the fetal period.

Man establishes the mechanism for eventual testicular descent during the embryonic period, retaining a column and core of undifferentiated mesenchyma between the testis and the future scrotum and passing through the abdominal wall, to be used later for testicular descent. This accomplished, there are few major changes until shortly before the time of testicular descent; therefore it is convenient to describe the process in two phases:

1. Establishment of the male reproductive system, transferring from the primitive common form when the testis produces testosterone. The female form is retained if testosterone production fails; male orientation develops in a genetic female if influenced by testosterone-like hormones.

2. Testicular descent much later in fetal life.

Both phases depend on production of testosterone by the testis under gonadotropic stimulation, although the source of the stimulus is still debatable, whether stemming from the maternal circulation, chorion, or fetal pituitary glands. There again appears to be a wide species variation; certain animals show a far more dramatic gonadotropic cutoff at birth, as evidenced by testicular activity, than others. In certain rodents (rat, mouse, California squirrel), the testes have descended to the small cremasteric sac by birth. Thereafter the sexual matur-

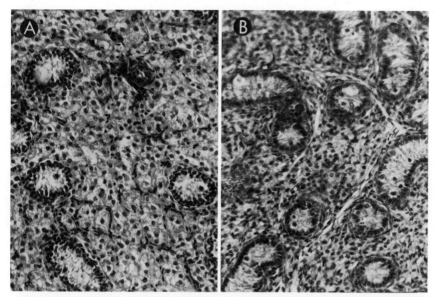

Fig 2–6. — Section of **(A)** a newborn seal testis and **(B)** four-day-old animal with a quarter testis weight. Picture is similar to but more dramatic than that of human early postpartum period.

ing process slows but nevertheless maintains a gradual development to early puberty, the large expansion and hypertrophy of the cremasteric sac followed by full descent of the testes into the sac. In certain circumstances the testes are returned to the abdomen by cremasteric contraction. In the gray seal at birth, there is a dramatic reduction in testicular bulk to a quarter of its birth weight in four days (Fig 2–6), largely at the expense of the interstitial tissue.

Presumably the seal shows an almost total dependence on maternal and/or placental gonadotropins. In man, although somewhat less dramatically, development resembles that of the seal more closely than it does that of the rodent.[19]

TESTICULAR DESCENT

As the time approaches for descent (at about seven months or later), a fairly rapid change occurs in the gubernaculum testis and associated structures. The gubernacular mesenchyma has retained its relatively primitive quality, but now begins to swell with the scrotum. No significant change in the number of cells appears, but the intercellular material increases enormously until it resembles Wharton's jelly in the postnatal umbilical cord. This intercellular material is rich in hyaluronic acid. The process takes place relatively slowly within the scrotum, causing the scrotal wall to dilate widely. We have shown in postnatal rats that hormonal stimulation alone will not greatly increase the size of the scrotum and cremasteric sacs at puberty; the mechanical effect of contained bulk must also be present. Under normal circumstances this is brought about by increased testicular and primarily epididymal bulk, e.g., in the sexually immature state before puberty, the cremasteric sac contains only the cauda epididymis. The sac dilates under the influence of the activating testis and appears to provide the primary bulk needed to initiate cremasteric hypertrophy. However, as this continues, both testis and epididymis become contained in the now large cremasteric sac. In our experimental model, we replaced the testis with a glass or stainless steel ball, which worked in a comparable way, but most effectively when the epididymis was retained to provide active contained bulk for the cremasteric swelling, as long as there was adequate testosterone replacement.

As stated above, it is important not to read too much into an interspecific study and in this case we were comparing an antenatal descent pattern with a postnatal one. Nevertheless, the enormous increase in gubernacular bulk within the scrotum appears, simply on the evidence of observation, to play an important part in the scrotal dilation taking place. In true cryptorchidism, the scrotum often remains small, without the normal stretched and wrinkled appearance seen in a retracted or ectopic testis.

With the marked increase in the gubernaculum bulk within the scrotum, a separation zone develops so that the large jelly-like gubernacular mass comes to lie free within the scrotum, i.e., it loses its attachment to the scrotal floor. This process is most obvious in the pig and ungulate fetuses in which the descent is apparently less rapid than in man (animal fetuses at this period in development are far easier to acquire than human ones for examination). Nevertheless, although the separation may precede testicular descent by a short time in man, it does occur unless there is evidence of a pathologic condition (Fig 2 – 7).

The increase in gubernacular bulk seen within the scrotum does not occur in the mesenchyma near the testis. Thus the once essentially cylindric gubernacular system becomes more conical or even piriform. Its dilating effect is primarily on the scrotum and to a lesser degree on the inguinal region.

Meanwhile, rapid changes occur in certain related structures. The processus vaginalis, which had shown minimal advancement distally,

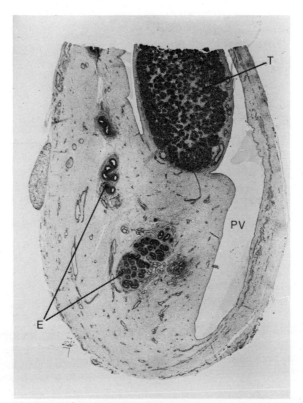

Fig 2–7. — Lower part of testis and gubernaculum of human fetus lifted out from completely separated scrotal wall shortly after descent. *T* = testis; *E* = epididymis; *PV* = processus vaginalis.

now actively invades the gubernacular mesenchyma into the scrotal region. The intra-abdominal gubernacular fold extends distally on a mesentery within the processus vaginalis into the scrotum, and the former peripheral part of the extra-abdominal gubernaculum is differentiated as a tube surrounding it.

The cremaster muscle likewise begins rapid growth and extends distally in the differentiated peripheral tube of the gubernaculum down into the scrotum. The muscle and processus vaginalis grow distally at about the same rate toward the tip of the gubernaculum. However, the cremaster muscles extend distally to produce their eventual anatomical form; the medial and lateral components spiral anteriorly, fibers crossing as they develop until they terminate at what eventually will be the root of the mesorchium, although at this time it is the distal root of the mesentery of the gubernacular fold.

The testis is now at the apex of an intraperitoneal gubernacular fold extending within the processus vaginalis in the inguinal region into the scrotum. The distal part of the fold will be markedly swollen, as is the distal part of the gubernaculum, and the portion close to the testis will be much narrower (Fig 2–8).

Up to this point there has been relatively little development of the extratesticular tubular system, the vas deferens, and the epididymis. The latter is rudimentary, with only a few coils in the proximal part of the gubernaculum. The blood vessels, testicular artery, and testicular venous complex also are relatively short, being essentially no longer than needed for the intra-abdominal testis. As the processus vaginalis and cremaster muscle burst into growth and activity, there also is rapid growth of the vas deferens and the blood vessels.

Although the gubernacular tip grows in bulk, considerably increasing the size of the scrotum, it grows far less in length or proximally in diameter. The gubernacular fold increases somewhat in length so that the distance from testis to scrotal floor increases slowly, but meanwhile the scrotum grows considerably, far more than the gubernacular length, so that it becomes relatively short compared with the scrotum and body wall. However, the peripheral part of the gubernaculum, which has been kept apart by the processus vaginalis and contains the cremaster muscle, also grows rapidly in much the same way as does the scrotal wall. It has virtually become body wall and grows with it now that it has differentiated from the central gubernacular mesenchyma. Thus as the body and scrotum grow (the latter probably influenced by the contained expanding gubernacular bulk), the gubernacular fold extending to the testis becomes relatively shorter and the fold also becomes more conical (see Fig 2–8). As both scrotum and inguinal canal are stretched by the gubernacular fold, their essentially conical shape, with the relatively small testes at the apex, allows the gonad to slip through the inguinal canal into the scrotum. Their downward progress is permitted by the rapid lengthening of the vas deferens and the testicular vessels. The actual descent process must be fairly rapid; among the considerable number of human, pig, and ungulate fetuses examined, the testis has been found in the canal only when an obvious mechanical factor such as a short artery prevents descent.

Several authors have held that the concept of gubernacular shortening in testicular descent is untenable[17, 20, 21] inasmuch as the gubernaculum grows faster than the body wall. This is of course true when the gubernaculum is measured only against the fetal body (i.e., C-R length) itself and prior to descent. This is substantiated by the fact that the huge increase in intercellular fluid, particularly in the scrotal re-

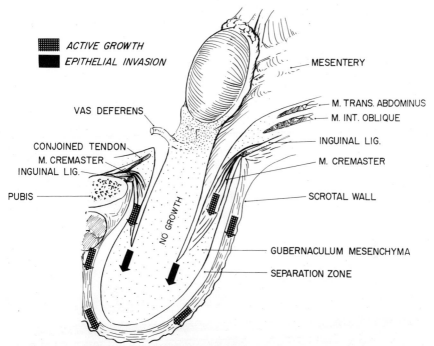

ACTIVE GROWTH
EPITHELIAL INVASION

MESENTERY

VAS DEFERENS

M. TRANS. ABDOMINUS
M. INT. OBLIQUE

CONJOINED TENDON
M. CREMASTER
INGUINAL LIG.

INGUINAL LIG.

M. CREMASTER

PUBIS

SCROTAL WALL

NO GROWTH

GUBERNACULUM MESENCHYMA

SEPARATION ZONE

Fig 2–8.—Diagrammatic representation of testis, gubernaculum, and changes occurring as descent approaches. Density of *dots* in gubernaculum indicates cell population in intercellular fluid.

gion, leads to greater gubernacular bulk, which also is reflected in its length. However, if the measurement includes the dilating scrotum, the growth differential is reversed and the shortening concept becomes fully tenable. Furthermore, with descent, the shortening process continues, allowing scrotal space for the growing testis and epididymis.

The role of intra-abdominal pressure in testicular descent has been postulated by Gier and Marion,[22] among others. Whatever other evidence is produced, the apparent speed of descent, once the conditions have been established, is the final motivating force, assisted possibly by the conical shape of the gubernacular fold within the lubricated processus vaginalis.

Rajfer and Walsh[21] postulate that "during the actual event of testicular descent the gubernaculum that is in contact with the testis degenerates, thus allowing the testis to migrate along the pathway of the disappearing gubernaculum." This view is difficult to accept without evidence of such paratesticular degeneration. In fact, this region does not become involved in the dilatation but remains more or less as it has throughout its development. This difference probably prompted their concept of degeneration. However, the postulate can be accepted in reverse, i.e., that the gubernaculum distally dilates the system and thereafter reduces in bulk by differentiation; this feature becomes more obvious subsequent to descent.

After descent the inguinal canal, which had been filled by the gubernacular plug, assumes a far more oblique and closed form of normal mature anatomy, although traversed by an open but narrow vaginal canal.

CHANGES FOLLOWING TESTICULAR DESCENT

Once the gubernaculum has swelled and the scrotum and inguinal canal have dilated, followed by passage of the testis through the canal, its large globular jelly-like tip, lying free in the scrotum, diminishes. This is in part due to a reduction in its length, allowing the testis to move nearer to the scrotal floor. In any case the distal gubernacular bulk was mainly in intercellular fluid. When the testis is contained in the scrotum (or even if the testis fails to descend), there is a marked reduction in this intercellular fluid, automatically leading to shortening as a component of reduced gubernacular bulk.

The tissue now begins to differentiate into the loose distal coverings of the testis (Fig 2–9). The processus vaginalis has completed its growth into the gubernacular tip. The surrounding tissues containing the cremaster muscle become the internal and external spermatic fasciae (Fig 2–10). What factors lead to these changes in the gubernaculum are perhaps more difficult to explain than the process of descent itself. The tremendous increase in intercellular fluid could be attributed to the same hormonal stimulii that influence the enormous growth of the vas deferens, epididymis, and testicular vessels. However, after the work of dilatation has been completed, with probable testicular descent, the interstitial tissue is reduced again and the mesenchymal cells of the gubernaculum differentiate toward fibroblasts. Perhaps the very burst of activity itself may trigger differentiation. The hormonal reduction with birth may be the partial cause, although the process begins after the testis has descended and may be well advanced at birth.

At the time of testicular descent, the epididymis remains as a few rudimentary loops, but as the vas deferens grows rapidly, allowing descent, this rapid lengthening continues, producing the coils of the

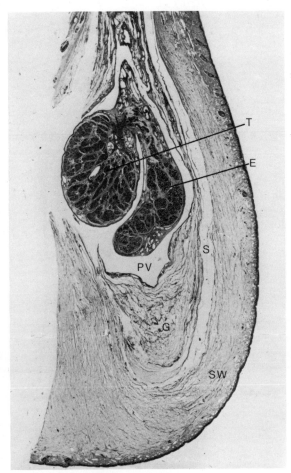

Fig 2–9.—Section through left scrotum containing testis *(T)*, epididymis *(E)*, with gubernacular remnant *(G)* now differentiating in near-term fetus. *PV* = processus vaginalis; *SW* = scrotal wall; *S* = separation zone between the gubernaculum and the scrotal wall.

epididymis, which develop in the gubernacular mesenchyma in the vicinity of the testes. With the growth of the epididymis, the last part of the gubernaculum also differentiates into the supporting epididymal fascia.

The gubernaculum testis can thus be described as a mass of mesenchyma that does not differentiate with the surrounding body structures. Instead it persists to prepare the way for testicular descent and

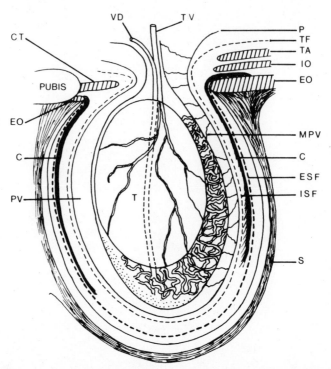

Fig 2–10.—Schematic representation of later gubernacular differentiation whose remnant is shown in *stipple,* containing the epididymis. *CT* = conjointed tendon; *VD* = vas deferens; *TV* = testicular vessels; *P* = peritoneum; *TF* = transversalis fascia; *TA* = transversus abdominis; *IO* = internal oblique; *EO* = external oblique; *PV* = processus vaginalis with its mesentery processus vaginalis (MPV); *C* = cremaster; *ESF* = external spermatic fascia; *ISF* = internal spermatic fascia; *S* = scrotal wall; *T* = testis.

remains as a medium into which the structures associated with the descending testis can differentiate at a much later stage of development than for most other structures.

That the process of testicular descent is directly influenced by testosterone produced by the testis itself, stimulated by gonadotropins, is incontrovertible. However, there is still doubt, in man at least, as to where the necessary gonadotropic influence is secreted and whether significant amounts come from the fetal pituitary. It would appear from the behavior of the interstitial cells following birth that most of it must come from maternal sources and placental sources that are lost at birth. Views on the character and extent of testicular activity after birth vary; the present consensus has been well summarized by Hadžiselimović,[23] who indicates that there is a small degree of Leydig cell activity in the first year after birth. Nevertheless, it may be said that testicular descent either occurred before birth or is on the point of so doing if descent is to occur naturally in view of the major gonadotropic cutoff with birth.

TESTICULAR MALDESCENT

From what has already been stated, failure of testicular descent is likely to stem from one of two causes: (1) a failure of the hormonal environment or (2) mechanical failure. Hormonal failure usually is believed to produce a cryptorchid state, and mechanical problems to cause ectopic testis, but such generalization is better avoided.

Hormonal Failure

Hormonal failure itself may occur in a variety of ways. It is debatable how much failure in gonadotropic stimulation affects failure of descent when pregnancy proceeds normally to full term. On the other hand, if the pregnancy is cut short by early parturition, then loss of gonadotropic stimulation may halt descent approximately to the extent that has occurred at parturition.

In other cases of obvious hormonal fault, it is harder to pinpoint the real cause. It can be shown in many cases of failure of descent that the testis remains small and apparently deficient in development. It is less easy to be certain whether the fault is in the gonadotropic stimulus or in the testicular development itself despite normal gonadotropic supply. Whatever the cause, in many cases there is failure of testicular interstitial activity, which in turn limits the changes required for normal testicular descent. Frequently a cryptorchid state appears to be due to a short artery or, less often, to a vein or vas deferens, which therefore prevents descent. Nevertheless, this may be owing to hormonal failure, for, as described above, the growth processes associated with descent include the rapid elongation of these structures. If the testis is obviously abnormal, it is reasonable to argue a case for hormonal deficiency, but when the testis appears more normal in development, the target organ may fail to grow in response to the hormone. For the moment there are many questions to be answered in this field.

Mechanical Failure

Although failure of descent due to a short artery or vas can be considered a mechanical failure, it is likely to be primarily hormonal. However, any interference with the normal anatomical development of the gubernaculum and associated structures can limit descent or produce another abnormality, usually of position. Indeed, any morphological abnormality in pelvic development might interfere with the normal development and movement of the testis and vas, thereby limiting descent. One well-known interrelationship is that between an abnormally placed (usually pelvic or horseshoe) kidney and an undescended testis. In the cases examined as fetuses in which this relationship existed, the gubernacular development appeared normal distally; the deficiency seemed to be one of a short vas deferens, presumably a lesion associated with a maldevelopment of the metanephric diverticulum of the mesonephric duct from which both developed. The vessels were, however, also short. In our two anomalies found in fetuses, the testes appeared normal for the stage of development and were comparable to those of the other side, which had descended normally; thus, we consider this form of maldescent to be mechanical due to a developmental rather than hormonal failure.

With respect to ectopia testis, Lockwood[24] described peripheral fibromuscular attachments of the gubernaculum to the possible ectopic sites as well as to the floor of the scrotum. Although this view is still commonly held to explain the condition, the normal gubernaculum is not a fibromuscular cord as described, and hence the various peripheral gubernacular attachments pulling the testis out of position must be dismissed. Nevertheless in ectopia testis, the fibrous bands attaching the testis to its abnormal site can be shown to exist. Lockwood dissected these bands in the fetus, and the original Lockwood dissection still exists in the Anatomy Museum of St. Bartholomew's Hospital. From this and from repeat dissections, it appears that what Lockwood dissected was the developing peripheral fascia around the gubernaculum. Because the latter is a simple, soft, jelly-like structure, it was probably dismissed as merely undifferentiated packing tissue or a central soft core of the presumed fibromuscular gubernaculum, an understandable mistake, especially in view of the very real fibrous bands of ectopia testis.

In the developing state, the gubernaculum must remain as an undifferentiated mesenchymatous mass into which the processus vaginalis and the cremaster muscle can grow and differentiate. It is important that as the body wall and scrotal fasciae differentiate in the fetus, the fibrous tissue and abdominal muscles not encroach on the gubernaculum. Encroachment of the developing fibrous tissue into the gubernacular mesenchyma will effectively prevent the downward growth of the processus vaginalis and the cremaster muscle at that site (Fig 2–11). In the remaining part of the gubernaculum, without invasion, their growth will occur normally. Although we have not found such invasion in human fetuses, we have observed it in pigs. Because the

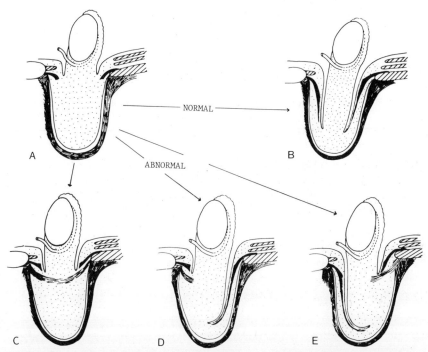

Fig 2–11. — Diagrammatic representation of normal **(A – B)** development of processus vaginalis and cremaster into gubernacular mesenchyma, presented in **C,** full septum, **D,** pubic, and **E,** superficial inguinal fibrous encroachment, which will thus produce fibrous "tails of Lockwood"[24] in ectopia testis.

pig is remarkably like man with respect to the overall pattern of the process, it appears reasonable to assume that the mechanism also is similar. It is easy to recognize that the pattern observed in the pig fetus leads to the morphological pattern of the human ectopic testis, which is comparable morphologically to the essential anatomy of a pig ectopic testis. A small invasion of fibrous tissue at one site will set up the fibrous band shown by Lockwood to form the necessary anchor for one or another of the peripheral sites of ectopia. These peripheral sites also provide the attachments of normal fascia. As the normal cremaster and processus vaginalis develop elsewhere in the gubernaculum (and with other changes such as normal swelling), the normal descent process is limited only by the fibrous band and the deficient processus vaginalis at that point. Thus the testis is free to descend normally but only as far as the anchor point. Because of this and the pattern of development of the processus vaginalis, the testis will swing out of the normal line of descent in much the same way as a boat tethered to the bank of a stream will be carried into the shore by the current.

From time to time cases are seen in which there is a complete barrier across the external ring, a continuation of the abdominal wall fascia below which there may be a relatively small, wrinkled, albeit empty scrotum. Such a condition can be explained as an extension of the small fibrous invasion of the ectopic testis entirely across the gubernaculum. The distal mesenchyma may still exist as a pocket that will allow normal scrotal development, but the testis will be totally blocked in its descent. If this explanation is correct, which seems likely according to the available evidence, such a condition should be grouped clinically with ectopia testis, i.e., a mechanical failure, although by definition, as with the other intra-abdominal mechanical failures, it is diagnosed as cryptorchid. Yet here, as with other mechanical failures, the hormonal environment (at least initially in the fetal period) appears normal. The secondary changes to be expected in an undescended testis will of course develop later from its abnormal position.

REFERENCES
1. Witschi E.: Migrations of the germ cells of human embryos from the yolk sac to the primitive gonadal folds. *Contrib. Embryol. Carneg. Inst.* 32:67, 1948.
2. Giroud A.: *La fonction spermatogénétique du testicule humain.* Paris, Masson, 1958.
3. Jost A.: *The Role of Fetal Hormones in Prenatal Development.* Harvey Lectures, ser. 55. New York and London, Academic Press, 1961.
4. Baillie A. H., Ferguson M.M., Hart D.M.: *Developments in Histochemistry.* New York, Academic Press, 1966.
5. Black V.H., Christensen A.K.: Differentiation of interstitial cells and Sertoli cells in fetal guinea pig testes. *Am. J. Anat.* 124:211, 1969.
6. Holstein A.F., Wartenberg H., Vossmeyer J.: Zur cytologie der pränatalan Gonadenentwicklung beim Menschen. *Z. Anat. Entwickl. Gesch.* 135:43, 1971.
7. Backhouse K.M., Butler H.: The gubernaculum testis of the pig (sus scrofa). *J. Anat.* 94:109, 1960.
8. Backhouse K.M.: The gubernaculum testis Hunteri: Testicular descent and maldescent. *Ann. R. Coll. Surg. Engl.* 35:15, 1964.
9. Hunter J.: Observations on the state of the testis in the foetus and on the hernia congenita, in Hunter W.: *Medical Commentaries,* part 1. London, A. Hamilton, 1762.
10. Seiler B.W.: *Observationes nonnulles de testiculorum ex abdomine in scrotum descensu et partium genitalium anomaliis.* Leipzig, 1817.
11. Backhouse K.M.: Testicular descent and ascent in mammals. *Proc. XV Internat. Cong. Zool.* London, 1959, p. 413.

12. Cloquet J.: *Recherches anatomiques sur les hernies de l'abdomen*. Paris, 1817.
13. Carus C.G.: *An Introduction to the Comparative Anatomy of Animals*. London, 1827.
14. Hollingshead W.H.: *Anatomy for Surgeons*. New York, Harper & Row, 1971, vol. 2.
15. Cunningham C.: In Romanes G.J. (ed.): *Textbook of Anatomy*. London, Oxford University Press, 1972.
16. Gray H.: In Gross C.M. (ed.): *Anatomy of the Human Body*. Philadelphia, Lea & Febiger, 1973.
17. Lemeh C.N.: A study of the development and structural relationships of the testis and gubernaculum. *Surg. Gynecol. Obstet.* 110:164, 1960.
18. Backhouse K.M.: The cremaster muscle and testicular descent. *Ann. R. Coll. Surg. Engl.* 61:315, 1979.
19. Backhouse K.M.: The natural history of testicular descent and maldescent. *Proc. R. Soc. Med.* 59:357, 1966.
20. Wyndham N.R.: A morphological study of testicular descent. *J. Anat.* 77:179, 1943.
21. Rajfer J., Walsh P.C.: Testicular descent: Normal and abnormal. *Urol. Clin. North Am.* 5:224, 1978.
22. Gier H.T., Marion G.B.: Development of the mammalian testis, in Johnson A.D., Gomes W.R., Van Demark L. (eds.): *The Testis*. New York, Academic Press, 1970, vol. 1, p. 1.
23. Hadžiselimović F.: Cryptorchidism. *Adv. Anat. Embryol. Cell. Biol.* 53:1, 1977.
24. Lockwood C.B.: Development and transition of the testis, normal and abnormal. *J. Anat. Physiol.* 21:635, 22:38, 461, 505, 1887–1888.

3 / The Gubernaculum and Testicular Descent

JAYANT RADHAKRISHNAN, M.D.
PATRICIA K. DONAHOE, M.D.

IN 1762 HUNTER[1] PROPOSED that the cord attaching the lower pole of the testis to the abdominal wall prepared a path for testicular descent. Likening its function to the guiding action of a ship's helm, he named the cord the gubernaculum testis. Over the past two centuries many investigators have noted that the gubernaculum is conspicuous during testicular descent but virtually disappears after completion of this process. However, its function in testicular descent remains an enigma.

Hart[2] speculated that differential growth of the lumbar region of the fetus caused transabdominal migration of the testis, whereas the gubernaculum remained essentially static. Gier and Marion[3] also believed that the gubernaculum played a passive role in testicular descent, that of showing the testis the direction it should follow; actual descent, they believed, resulted from intra-abdominal pressure. Wensing and Colenbrander[4] proposed that the swollen, unattached gubernaculum produced traction in the manner of a balloon passing through a tight ring, whereas Sonneland[5] suggested that the gubernaculum produced active traction by its muscular contractions. It is probable that all of these factors are involved to varying degrees in the complex process of testicular descent. It is our purpose, however, to describe morphological changes that occur in the gubernaculum while the testis is undergoing descent and to consider the hypothesis that spiral contractions of the gubernaculum create tension on the testis to cause its descent.

There is almost no agreement in the literature regarding the morphological character of the gubernaculum, a fact probably related to the stage of embryonic development at which the gubernaculum has been described by the various authors. Backhouse[6] described the gubernacular bulb as a free, jelly-like mass unattached to the abdominal wall. Elger et al.[7] and Tayakkanonta[8] reported that the gubernaculum testis consisted of striated muscle, and Tayakkononta[8] also showed that it had a rich nerve supply.

IN VIVO STUDIES

We studied the structure of the male and female fetal gubernaculum on sequential days using timed pregnant rats sacrificed from gestational day 14½, when gonadal sex can be differentiated, through day 21½, the last day of gestation. The gubernaculi of postnatal rats also were studied from day one to adulthood.[9] The gross anatomy of the pelvic and inguinal areas was examined (Fig 3–1) and photographed in situ. Most of the specimens were fixed in paraffin and stained with hematoxylin and eosin or Masson's stain. Selected specimens were fixed in 4% glutaraldehyde, osmificated, and embedded in Epon; 1-μ thick sections were then cut on a Porter-Blume microtome and stained with toluidine blue for light microscopy (Figs 3–2 and 3–3).

The gubernaculum of the 14½-day-old male embryo consisted of a cord and a bulb (see Fig 3–1, A). At this time the testis was high in the abdominal cavity, the gubernacular cord was long, and the bulb was not well developed. As pregnancy progressed, the testis moved downward and the gubernacular cord shortened (see Fig 3–1, B). Subsequently the gubernacular bulb increased in size, assuming the proportions of the testis itself by the 20th day of pregnancy (see Fig 3–1, C), at which time a clear space (the future processus vaginalis) around the anteroinferior portion of the gubernacular bulb also was noted. At birth, when the testis had descended to the lower inguinal canal, the gubernacular cord was extremely short and the bulb well developed. Immediately after birth (see Fig 3–1, D) the bulb became smaller as it migrated and was incorporated into the abdominal wall musculature at the site of formation of the future scrotum. Seven to 10 days after birth, the scrotum was well developed and descent of the testis was completed.

Before day 18 of gestation, the histologic appearance of the gubernacular bulb (see Fig 3–2, A) consisted primarily of indifferent, loose, round mesenchymal cells. Between days 18 and 20 of gestation, the bulb became more dense. The loose, round mesenchymal cells in the periphery of the bulb condensed, diminshed the intracellular spaces, and took on an elongated fibrillar configuration, converting first to myoblasts (see Figs 3–2, A, and 3–3, A) and then to rhabdomyoblasts (see Figs 3–2, B, and 3–3, B). The center of the bulb retained the

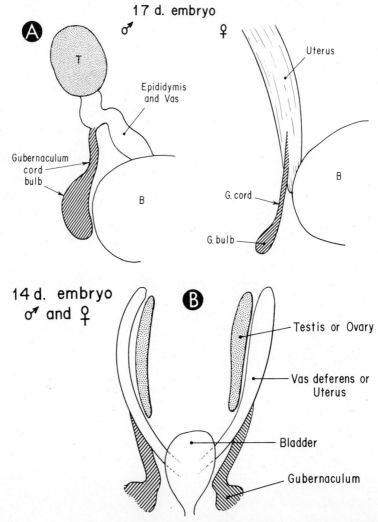

Fig 3–1.—A through **D,** diagrammatic representation of differentiation of gubernaculum in male and female rat fetuses at days 14, 17, and 20 of gestation, and one day after birth. *(Continued)*

loose mesenchymal form. By day 21 of gestation, the periphery of the gubernacular bulb thickened and differentiated from rhabdomyoblasts into cords of striated muscle (see Figs 3–2, C, and 3–3, C), which assumed a spiral configuration. By the second day of the postnatal period, the gubernacular bulb could no longer be detected.

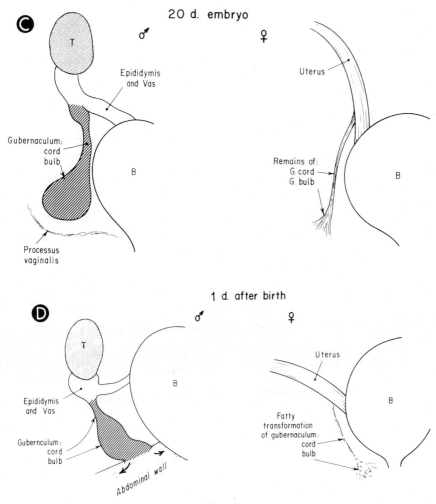

Fig 3–1.—(Cont.)

In the female the anatomy (see Fig 3–1) was almost identical to that of the male at day 14½. Between days 14½ and 17 (see Fig 3–1, B), the gubernaculum developed in essentially the same manner as that of the male, although the bulb never attained the same size. However, after day 17 the gubernacular bulb underwent progressive fatty metamorphosis (see Fig 3–1, C and D), which continued until the adult fatty, round ligament formed in the early postnatal period. Histologically the bulb of the female gubernaculum resembled the male guber-

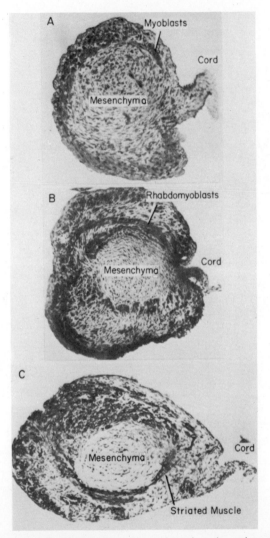

Fig 3–2.—**A** through **C,** photomicrographs of male gubernaculum at 18 days (×300), 20 days (×150), and 21 days (×130). Mesenchymal cells occupy center. Sequential differentiation of myoblasts **(A)** to striated muscle **(C)** is shown in periphery (1μ).

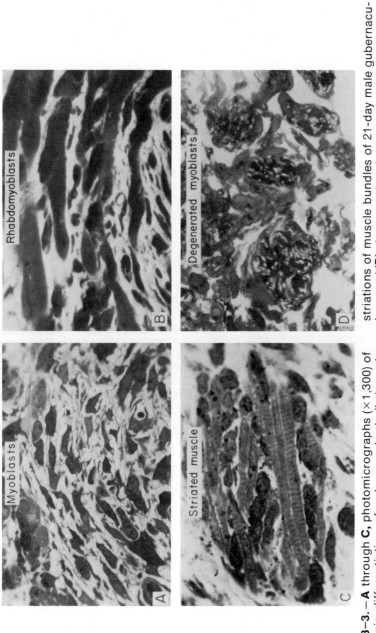

Fig 3–3. — **A** through **C**, photomicrographs (×1,300) of myogenic differentiation of gubernacular bulb in male embryo. **(A)**, myoblast of 18-day male gubernaculum; **(B)**, rhabdomyoblast of 20-day male gubernaculum; **(C)**, striations of muscle bundles of 21-day male gubernaculum; and **(D)**, degenerative changes in female gubernacular bulb at 18 days (1μ).

naculum until 18 days of gestation. The loose, round mesenchymal cells of the smaller female structure differentiated into elongated fibrillar cells in the periphery, but the circumferential layer was smaller than that of the male, and striations never developed. These cords of rhabdomyoblasts later underwent degeneration (see Fig 3–3, D) and were replaced by fat.

Thus in the male we found that the mesenchymal cells of the gubernacular bulb first developed into fibrillar cells, myoblasts, in the periphery (see Figs 3–2, A, and 3–3, A). These then thickened into rhabdomyoblasts (see Figs 3–2, B, and 3–3, B), which subsequently differentiated into striated muscle (see Figs 3–2, C, and 3–3, C). This occurred when testicular descent was most rapid. It is probable that the large body of peripheral striated muscle, rather than disappearing,[4] may migrate distally and fan outward into the presumptive dartos muscle of the scrotum. Further, it is important to note that sharp dissection was required in the present experiments to separate the gubernaculum bulb from the abdominal wall posteriorly and inferiorly. These findings are in contrast to those of Backhouse[6] and of Wensing and Colenbrander,[4] who believe that the gubernacular bulb has no attachment. It is significant that the longitudinal and circumferential striated muscle bundles are prominent when the gubernaculum is most prominent and the testis is undergoing maximal descent. Moreover the gubernacular bulb is attached to the point on the abdominal wall that would eventually develop into the scrotum. Certain structure-function relationships are implied by this arrangement, supporting the proposal that spiral gubernacular contractions create tension on the testis and induce its descent.

IN VITRO STUDIES

Ever since Engle[10] was able to induce testicular descent in monkeys by injecting an extract from urine of pregnant monkeys, investigators have been attempting to identify the responsible hormone(s). In our laboratories we failed to induce morphological changes in the gubernacular tissue in vitro by using whole testis, testosterone, or crude extracts with biologic activity for müllerian inhibiting substance.[11]

Testosterone in concentrations ranging from 10^{-6} to 10^{-5} μg/ml was added to the media beneath the 20-day-old male gubernaculum placed in organ culture to determine if the steroid would initiate differentiation of rhabdomyoblasts to striated muscle in vitro, as observed in vivo. We found that 10^{-5} μg/ml was toxic to the tissue and 10^{-6} gm/ml stimulated the wolffian duct in the fetal urogenital ridge. We therefore used 10^{-6} μg/ml in subsequent experiments. Gubernaculi also were co-cultured in vitro with fragments of whole fetal testis or with maternal muscle fragments as controls. The gubernaculi of 17-day-old female fetuses were similarly studied to determine if morphological changes in the male could be induced in vitro, and if fatty degeneration could be prevented. Crude extracts of bovine calf testis with biologic activity for müllerian inhibiting substance were added to the media of the organ culture dish in which the 20-day-old fetal male and the 17-day-old fetal female gubernaculi were cultured for 24, 48, or 72 hours.

Bovine calf testes were obtained from animals immediately after death and diced rapidly with an automatic tissue chopper. The minced tissue was extracted in 1 M guanidine hydrochloride with 5 mM benzamidine for 48 hours at 4 C with gentle stirring. The suspension was then ultracentrifuged for one hour at 4 C, dialyzed against distilled water overnight, against 1 M sodium chloride for 8 hours, and against continuous 0.15 mole sodium chloride pH 7.20 overnight.[11] The dialysate was then concentrated on an Amicon ultrafilter fitted with a PM 10 membrane to 20-ml volume. The retained solution, in 1-ml aliquots, which had caused regression of the müllerian ducts in an organ culture bioassay,[12] was mixed 1:1 with media [CMRL with 10% fetal calf serum, 1% penicillin (10,000 units/ml), and 1% streptomycin (10,000 μg/ml)], and 2 ml of the mixture placed in the well of an organ culture dish (Falcon 3010). The gubernaculum was dissected from the 17-day-old female embryo (N = 20) or the 20-day-old male embryo (N = 16) and placed on a stainless steel grid coated with a thin layer of 2% agar and incubated for 24, 48, or 72 hours at 37 C in 5% CO_2 and 95% air over the culture media. Gubernaculi were oriented, fixed in glutaraldehyde, osmificated, and embedded in Epon. One-micron sections were cut on a Porter-Blume microtome and stained with toluidine blue for light microscopy.

DISCUSSION

Neither whole testis fragments, testosterone, nor bovine testis extracts with biologic activity for müllerian inhibiting substance in the concentrations tested could induce morphological changes in the gubernaculum in vitro. Dihydrotestosterone (DHT) has not been tested in this system. Failure of response could be due to many factors. It may be that increased concentrations of müllerian inhibiting substance are necessary to induce a change, or that longitudinal tension may be required before morphological differentiation to striated muscle can occur. The scarcity of material with high biologic activity for müllerian inhibiting substance limited the number of studies that

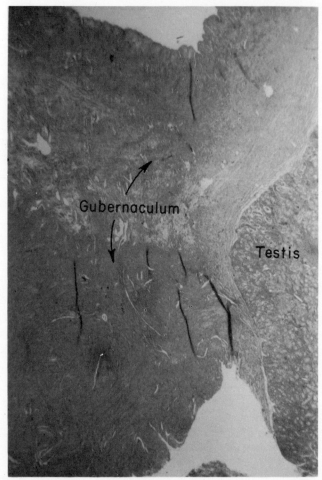

Fig 3–4.—Intra-abdominal testis and thickened fibrous gubernaculum from patient with testicular feminization.

could be performed. As more purified and concentrated material becomes available, more specific receptor studies can be done to investigate which hormonal factors control testicular descent. Recently, Rajfer and Walsh[13] have convincingly implicated DHT, finding that gonadotropin treatment or DHT (but not androstenedione or testosterone) replacement accelerated descent of the testis from an inguinal to a scrotal position in postnatal rats. In addition, inhibition of postnatal testicular descent in rats by estradiol was reversed by using DHT but not testosterone. They proposed that DHT mediated testicular descent and that gonadotropins were necessary to induce the testicular enzyme, 5α-reductase, to convert testosterone to DHT. Dihydrotestosterone studies should therefore be performed in vitro using the 20-day male fetal gubernaculum to determine whether, at this stage of fetal development, gubernaculum differentiation to striated muscle can be induced. Whole testis fragments may have been ineffective in this in vitro study if, as Rajfer and Walsh have shown in postnatal rats, gonadotropin stimulation is required to convert testosterone to DHT. It is of interest that men with testicular feminization syndrome who lack androgen receptors often have intra-abdominal testes with thick, fibrous gubernaculi, as seen in Figure 3–4; such gubernaculi may not undergo differentiation due to lack of androgen receptors.

The increased frequency of undescended testis in patients with Kallman's syndrome[14] (hypogonadotropic hypogonadism with anosmia) and the impaired LH response of cryptorchid children to LH-releasing hormone (LH-RH) stimulation[15] indicates that, although gonadotropins play a vital role in testicular descent, ultimate descent is mediated through the testis.

We suspect that one of the testicular hormones (testosterone, DHT, or müllerian inhibiting substance) may be necessary to modulate testicular descent and that the gubernaculum may be the receptor organ that responds to one of these hormones by differentiating into striated muscle that contracts to induce testicular descent. The fact that cryptorchidism is more commonly unilateral than bilateral makes it likelier that descent is related to locally active factors from the ipsilateral gonad rather than to generalized factors, e.g., increased intra-abdominal pressure, which would affect both gonads. Conversely, it is also interesting that in more generalized myogenic defects such as prune belly syndrome[16] or arthrogryposis (personal observations), maldescent is bilateral.

Short and colleagues[17, 18] have analyzed Saanen intersex goats, which have 60 XX female genotypes but male phenotypes except for the absence of horns (polled). This "experiment of nature" indicates that an autosome for hornlessness is associated with, or controls, sex determination, since these genetic females have azoospermic testes or ovatestes, as well as varying degrees of development of a male type of reproductive tract. Intersex goats often have gonadal asymmetry with a descended testis on one side and an undescended testis on the other. Interestingly, although Short et al.[17, 18] demonstrated that both testes of the intersex goats could produce testosterone, the undescended testis frequently was associated with retained müllerian duct structures and the descended testis with absent müllerian duct structures. This coincidence of events in the Saanen intersex goat might implicate müllerian inhibiting substance in descent of the testis.

Recently, Sloan and Walsh[19] and Brook et al.[20] described sibs with retained müllerian duct structures in an otherwise normal male phenotype. All of these individuals, however, also had undescended testes. Pappis et al.[21] described three unrelated infants with persistent müllerian ducts, with vas deferens entering the wall of the persistent uterine structures, each of whom also had bilateral undescended testes. A more recent study of the human testis[22] observed that müllerian inhibiting substance activity was lower in boys with undescended testes than in children with normal or intersex descended testes at comparable ages under two years.

If the testis is dysgenic, as in cases of dysgenic male pseudohermaphroditism[23] or mixed gonadal dysgenesis,[24] testicular descent does not occur. Hunter[25] questioned whether the testis became abnormal because it failed to descend or failed to descend because it was abnormal. We suspect that the latter is the case, except in rare myogenic disorders or in certain cases of gonadal deficiency attributable to hypothalamic or pituitary deficiency.[14] Considerable research remains to be done to elucidate all the mechanisms controlling testicular descent. If indeed the gubernaculum is a receptor organ responsible for descent of the testis, then its response to hormonal manipulation can be studied either in vivo or in vitro, with possible implications for the eventual management of undescended testes.

REFERENCES

1. Hunter J.: Observations on the state of the testis in the foetus and on the hernia congenita, in Hunter W.: *Medical Commentaries*, part 1. London, A. Hamilton, 1762, p. 75.
2. Hart D.B.: The nature and cause of the physiological descent of the testis. *J. Anat. Physiol.* 43:263, 1909.
3. Gier H.T., Marion G.B.: Development of the mammalian testis, in Johnson A.D., Gomes W.R., Van Demark L. (eds.): *The Testis*, New York, Academic Press, 1970, vol 1, p. 1.
4. Wensing C.J., Colenbrander B.: The process of normal and abnormal testicular descent, in Bierich J.R.: *Maldescensus Testis*. Baltimore, Urban and Schwarzenberg, 1977, p. 193.
5. Sonneland S.G.: Congenital perineal testicle. *Ann. Surg.* 80:716, 1924.
6. Backhouse K.M.: The gubernaculum testis hunteri: Testicular descent and maldescent. *Ann. R. Coll. Surg. Engl.* 35:15, 1964.
7. Elger W., Richter J., Korte R.: Failure to detect androgen dependence of the descensus testiculorum in foetal rabbits, mice and monkeys, in *Maldescensus Testis*. Baltimore, Urban and Schwarzenberg, 1977, p. 187.
8. Tayakkanonta K.: The gubernaculum testis and its nerve supply. *Aust. N.Z. J. Surg.* 33:61, 1963.

9. Radhakrishnan J., Morikawa Y., Donahoe P.K., et al.: Observations on the gubernaculum during descent of the testis. *Invest. Urol.* 16:365, 1979.
10. Engle E.T.: Experimentally induced descent of the testis in the macaque monkey by hormones from the anterior pituitary and pregnancy urine. *Endocrinology* 16:513, 1932.
11. Swann D.A., Donahoe P.K., Ito Y., et al.: Extraction of müllerian inhibiting substance from newborn calf testis. *Dev. Biol.* 69:73, 1979.
12. Donahoe P.K., Ito Y., Hendren W.H.: A graded organ culture assay for the detection of müllerian inhibiting substance. *J. Surg. Res.* 23:141, 1977.
13. Rajfer J., Walsh P.C.: Hormonal regulation of testicular descent: Experimental and clinical observations. *J. Urol.* 118:985, 1977.
14. Kallman F.J., Schoenfeld W.A., Barrera S.E.: The genetic aspects of primary eunuchoidism. *Am. J. Ment. Defic.* 48:203, 1974.
15. Job J.C., Garnier P.E., Chaussain J.L., et al.: Effect of synthetic LH-RH on the release of gonadotropins in hypophysogonadal disorders in children and adolescents. IV. Undescended testes. *J. Pediatr.* 84:371, 1974.
16. Williams D.I., Burkholder G.: The prune belly syndrome. *J. Urol.* 98:244, 1967.
17. Short R.V., Hamerton J.L., Grieves S.A., et al.: An intersex goat with a bilaterally asymmetrical reproductive tract. *J. Reprod. Fertil.* 16:283, 1968.
18. Short R V.: An introduction to some problems of intersexuality. *J. Reprod. Fertil.* 16:283, 1968.
19. Sloan W.R., Walsh P.C.: Familial persistent müllerian duct syndrome. *J. Urol.* 115:459, 1976.
20. Brook C.G.D., Wagner H., Zachman M.: Familial occurrence of persistent müllerian structures in otherwise normal males. *Br. Med. J.* 1:771, 1973.
21. Pappis C., Constantinides C., Chiotis D., et al.: Persistent müllerian duct structures in cryptorchid male infants: Surgical dilemmas. *J. Pediatr. Surg.* 14:128, 1979.
22. Donahoe P.K., Ito Y., Morikawa Y., et al.: Müllerian inhibiting substance in human testes after birth. *J. Pediatr. Surg.* 12:323, 1977.
23. Donahoe P.K., Crawford J.D., Hendren W.H.: Management of neonates and children with male pseudohermaphroditism. *J. Pediatr. Surg.* 12:1045, 1977.
24. Donahoe P.K., Crawford J.D., Hendren W.H.: Mixed gonadal dysgenesis, pathogenesis, and management. *J. Pediatr. Surg.* 14:287, 1979.
25. Hunter J.: Description of the situation of the testis in the foetus with its descent into the scrotum, in *The Complete Works of John Hunter F.R.S.* Philadelphia, Palmer, 1841, p. 41.

4 / Incidence of Testicular Maldescent

ERIC W. FONKALSRUD, M.D.

TRUE CRYPTORCHIDISM represents a congenital arrest of the normal descent of the testis into the scrotum. Scorer[1] personally surveyed more than 3,500 newborn males and found 4.3% with undescended testes. The occurrence of cryptorchidism was 2.7% in full-term infants (weighing more than 2,500 gm) and 21% in premature infants. A similar incidence of maldescent in full-term and premature infants was recorded by Hofstatter[2] in 1912. As great as 10% of newborn males were recorded by Bishop[3] in 1945 as having testicular undescent. Neonatologists, however, indicate that the testes are descended in more than 99% of newborn full-term males and that retraction up into the inguinal canal occurs only after the first few weeks of life in most cases. Detailed analyses of available statistics indicate a direct correlation between the degree of prematurity and the frequency of undescent. Infants with a birth weight under 1,500 gm have a 60–70% incidence of cryptorchidism. However, the correlation of undescent tends to parallel the gestational age rather than the actual birth weight, since the testes do not begin their descent into the scrotum until the eighth month of embryonal development.

Scorer[4] noted that two thirds of the undescended testes in full-term males at birth eventually descended into a normal position in the scrotum by six weeks of age (three months for premature infants). If descent did not occur by this time, the testis never descended completely and remained smaller than the contralaterally descended gonad. Other authors have observed that as many as 2% of males at age one year have cryptorchidism but that this figure decreases to 1% at puberty.[3, 5] Scorer[1] found that only 28 of 3,612 boys (0.8%) examined at age one year had one or both testes remaining undescended, probably representing the true incidence of undescended testes in boyhood. In almost half of these boys, the testis was located in a high scrotal position, a condition that many other authors may not have classified as cryptorchidism; this then concurs with the more commonly observed incidence of complete undescent approximating 0.4% if the high scrotal gonads are omitted.

A recent statistical review by Buemann et al.[6] from Sweden indicates that the incidence of undescent at age one year in 20,000 children was 1% to 1.8%, similar to that presented by Scorer. The figure of 0.8% with undescent also was noted by Cour-Palais[7] in 4,680 boys screened by him personally. In the largest statistical review of the subject, Campbell[8] in 1959 reported that cryptorchidism occurred in 0.44% of adult males, based on 2.8 million United States Selective Service physical examinations between 1940 and 1944. Baumrucker[9] recorded an incidence of 0.75% for 10,000 consecutive inductees into the U.S. Army during World War II. It is difficult to determine accurately the incidence of undescended testes in the general population because most authors do not clearly specify what is meant by nondescent, i.e., at what level in the scrotum the testis is considered descended.

Scorer[1, 10] further emphasized that the testis must reside in or be capable of manipulation into a position more than 8 cm below the pubic crest in order to be considered normally descended. Gonads that cannot be manipulated lower than 3–6 cm below the pubic tubercle have been classified as "incompletely descended" even though they may eventually reside in the high scrotum. These gonads usually are smaller than normal descended testes of the male of the same age. An analysis of the final position of the testes in 100 consecutive children with undescent is shown in Table 4–1, which indicates that 48% had incompletely descended testes. Like the more typical true undescended testes, incompletely descended testes frequently are associated with an inguinal hernia, since the processus vaginalis usually closes completely only when the testis has reached its point of full descent.[11]

About 14% of boys with undescended testes come from families in

TABLE 4–1.—ANALYSIS OF FINAL POSITION IN 100
DYSTOPIC TESTES°

LOCATION	RIGHT	LEFT	
Absent, abdominal, or undetermined	5	6	
In inguinal canal	7	10	52%
In superficial inguinal pouch	16	8	
Incompletely descended (in high scrotum)	25	23	48%
Total	53	47	

°In 10 children nondescent was bilateral. (Adapted from Scorer.[1])

which other members have the same condition, although the mode of transmission is not yet known.[12] Perrett and O'Rourke[13] described eight cases of cryptorchidism in four generations, and there are many other reports of occurrence among brothers or in father and son.[14]

Most physicians who provide medical care for children believe that cryptorchid testes often will descend spontaneously when a boy passes through puberty into adolescence. Johnson,[15] who has been cited frequently, reported in 1939 that he had examined 31,609 boys in New York and found 544 cases of undescended testes (1.7%). Among these boys, 217 were lost to follow up, 14 were operated on, and spontaneous descent occurred in 313. A similar incidence of spontaneous descent was noted by Ward and Hunter[16] based on annual school examinations of 19,000 children in Nottingham, England. Unfortunately, no definition was provided to indicate what constituted an undescended testis, and the examinations were performed by many physicians. Scorer[1] suggested that this series probably included a large number of children with retractile testes, since almost half were reported to have bilateral undescent. It is also likely that many who were classified as having spontaneous descent at puberty had incompletely descended testes that came to lie in the upper scrotum. No clear evidence exists that the hormonal influences occurring at puberty, causing enlargement of the testes and external genitalia and decreasing the muscular pull of the cremaster, have any effect on the embryologic migration of the true cryptorchid gonad from the abdomen or inguinal canal. Thus, contrary to previous recommendations, there is no valid reason to defer the surgical management of true undescended testes until puberty.

The reported incidence of bilateral undescent has varied from 10%[17] to 25%[18] in two large series of boys operated on for cryptorchidism. The right side is undescended slightly more often (53–58%)[1] than the left (42–47%).[19]

REFERENCES
1. Scorer C.G.: The descent of the testis. *Arch. Dis. Child.* 39:605, 1964.
2. Hofstatter R.: Uber Kryptorchismus und Anomalien der Descenses testiculi. *Klin. Jahrb.* 26:155, 1912.
3. Bishop P.M.F.: Studies in clinical endocrinology: Management of the undescended testicle. *Guy's Hosp. Rep.* 94:12, 1945.
4. Scorer C.G.: The incidence of incomplete descent of the testicle at birth. *Arch. Dis. Child.* 31:198, 1956.
5. Nelson W.O.: Some problems of testicular function. *J. Urol.* 69:325, 1953.
6. Buemann B., Henriksen H., Villuhsen A.L., et al.: Incidence of undescended testis in the newborn. *Acta Chir. Scand.* 283[suppl.]:289, 1961.
7. Cour-Palais I.J.: Spontaneous descent of the testicle. *Lancet* 1:403, 1966.

8. Campbell H.E.: The incidence of malignant growth of the undescended testicle — a reply and re-evaluation. *J. Urol.* 81:663, 1959.
9. Baumrucker G.O.: Incidence of testicular pathology. *Bull. U.S. Army M. Dept.* 5:312, 1946.
10. Scorer C.G.: Descent of the testis in the first year of life. *Br. J. Surg.* 27:374, 1955.
11. Scorer C.G.: The anatomy of testicular descent — normal and incomplete. *Br. J. Surg.* 49:357, 1962.
12. Scorer C.G., Farrington G.H.: *Congenital Deformities of the Testis and Epididymis.* New York, Appleton-Century-Crofts, 1971.
13. Perrett L.J., O'Rourke D.A.: Hereditary cryptorchidism. *Med. J. Aust.* 1:1289, 1969.
14. Corbus B.C., O'Connor V.J.: The familial occurrence of undescended testis. *Surg. Gynecol. Obstet.* 34:237, 1922.
15. Johnson W.W.: Cryptorchidism. *J.A.M.A.* 113:25, 1939.
16. Ward B., Hunter W.M.: The absent testicle; a report on a survey carried out among school boys in Nottingham. *Br. Med. J.* 5179:110, 1960.
17. Snyder W.H. Jr., Chaffin L.: Surgical management of undescended testes. *J.A.M.A.* 157:129, 1955.
18. Gross R.E., Jewett T.C. Jr.: Surgical experience from 1222 operations for undescended testes. *J.A.M.A.* 160:634, 1956.
19. Mack W.S., Scott L.S., Ferguson-Smith M.A., et al.: Ectopic testis and true undescended testis: A histological comparison. *J. Pathol.* 82:439, 1961.

5 / Types of Testicular Maldescent

ERIC W. FONKALSRUD, M.D.

AN EMPTY SCROTUM may be the result of truly undescended, retractile, ectopic, atrophic, or absent testes. In 1955, Hinman[1] described three categories of undescended testes. The first, which includes physical abnormalities of the gubernaculum or inguinal canal leading to obstructed descent of an otherwise normal testis, accounts for most patients with an empty scrotum who require surgical care. The remaining chapters of this book are primarily concerned with this anomaly. The second type is the dysgenic testis, which is itself grossly and histologically abnormal and usually situated high in the inguinal canal or in the retroperitoneal space or sometimes is completely atrophic. The third category comprises patients with primary endocrine abnormalities in whom pituitary hypofunction fails to provide the hormonal stimulus necessary for testicular descent during and after gestation.

To supplement Hinman's classification, a fourth type of maldescent is the ectopic testis, which lies out of the path of normal descent, outside the external inguinal ring, usually in the suprapubic area or in the perineum. Finally, and of particular importance, the retractile testis is perhaps the most common cause of an empty scrotum in the prepubertal male, and requires careful identification by the physician to avoid unnecessary surgical repair.

DIAGNOSIS OF CRYPTORCHIDISM

Any male with an empty scrotum should be suspected of being cryptorchid. Although some parents are poor historians when it comes to observation of their son's scrotum, the majority will be able to indicate with certainty that the testis has or has not been present in the scrotum at some time since birth. Often the parents will have observed that the testis descends into the scrotum when the boy is taking a warm bath or sleeping, and then retracts into the inguinal canal when stimulated. Careful examination of the abdomen, inguinal re-

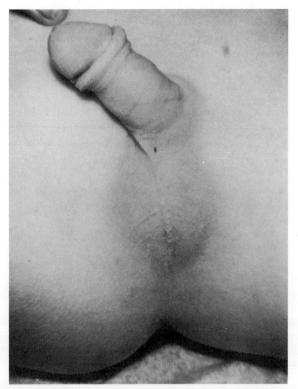

Fig 5–1.—Undeveloped and poorly rugated scrotum in five-year-old boy with bilateral high inguinal cryptorchid testes. (From Fonkalsrud, E.W., *Curr. Probl. Surg.* 15:1, 1978. Used with permission.)

gion, perineum, and scrotum by the physician, with warm hands, while the patient is relaxed in a recumbent position with knees elevated, usually enables identification of the testes. In over 85% of patients, the gonad can be felt at the level of the external inguinal ring or along the course of the inguinal canal. An undeveloped, poorly rugated scrotum is uncommon and, when present, usually occurs in association with a high inguinal or abdominal testis, or with an atrophic or absent gonad (Fig 5–1).

When the gonad is identified in a suprascrotal position, notation should be made not only regarding the size compared to the contralateral gonad and the gonads of other males of the same age, but also regarding the shape and consistency of the testis. After palpation, the fingers of the examining hand are pressed flat against the patient's lower abdomen just superior to the gonad and then slowly brought downward over the external inguinal ring with a sweeping motion in an attempt to manipulate the testis downward into the scrotum. The fingers of the other hand may assist by grasping the testis when it passes the scrotal neck and directing it into the scrotum as far as possible. This maneuver is repeated several times while noting the lowermost location in which the testis can be positioned, e.g., low inguinal canal, superficial inguinal pouch, high scrotum, or low scrotum (normal).[2] If the gonad cannot be manipulated into the scrotum, further examination of the patient in a standing or sitting position with the legs crossed may cause the testis to descend slightly lower. Occasionally, mild sedation may be necessary to facilitate an optimal examination of a hyperactive or unusually "ticklish" child.

If, in a given case, the testis cannot be felt anywhere, dogmatic statements regarding "absence" should not be made after a single examination.[3] On rare occasions, a high testis can momentarily slide up the canal into the abdomen and elude detection. Repeated examinations may be required in such cases to identify the testis when it retracts through the internal inguinal ring.[4] If, after several examinations, the physician is unable to palpate a testis, it probably is located in the abdomen, or it may be atrophic or absent. A large inguinal lymph node sometimes deceives the examiner into believing that a testis is present, although nodes tend to be inferior to the inguinal ligament, superficial, and multiple. Identification of an undescended testis may be particularly difficult in an obese child.

When the testis cannot be palpated, additional studies should be performed to determine if a gonad is present and to further define the location. A diagnostic course of human chorionic gonadotropin (HCG) (2,000 units intramuscularly every other day for five doses) may be helpful in distinguishing a true cryptorchid testis from a retractile testis that cannot be easily manipulated into the scrotum. In patients with bilateral undescent, a course of HCG, with measurements of plasma testosterone levels prior to and following the injections, will indicate by a rise in these levels whether Leydig cells and thus testes are present. It is clear that HCG will cause a rapid increase in vascular flow, vessel size, and maturation of the testis, but there is no indication that the short spermatic artery, which is the limiting factor in most cryptorchid testes, will be lengthened significantly by hormone treatment. Gross and Replogle,[5] Rea,[6] and many others call attention to the fact that generally the "successful" results following hormone administration have been achieved in boys who had retractile testes that subsequently would have descended spontaneously when endogenous gonadotropic hormones were produced in sufficient quantity.

These authors point out that the true cryptorchid testis is mechanically anchored in its downward pathway and that this obstacle cannot be overcome by exogenous administration of hormones. Lattimer et al.[7] believe that HCG may be helpful in enlarging the seriously underdeveloped scrotum before orchiopexy. Others suggest a trial of HCG for almost all patients with bilateral undescent and for those with unilateral undescent in whom obstructing mechanical factors are not believed to be present.[8] Thompson and Heckel[9] conclude that gonadotropins cause descent only of those testes that ultimately would have descended without treatment. They advocate hormone administration merely as a method of distinguishing testes that are destined to descend spontaneously from those that will require orchiopexy. They also point out that gonadotropin administration, even when it fails to cause descent, enlarges the testes and thus facilitates subsequent surgery. Further discussion regarding the use of HCG in the management of undescended testes is presented in Chapters 14 and 15.

Diagnostic ultrasound and/or computerized axial tomography (CAT) scans may be helpful in identifying abdominal testes and have the advantage of being noninvasive techniques, although experience has been limited. White et al.[10] were able to locate the cryptorchid testes in 80% of their patients by transperitoneal herniography. Selective arteriography,[11] venography,[12] and retroperitoneal pneumography also have been described as techniques for locating abdominal testes. Examination for radioactive ^{32}P uptake over the testis with scintiscans has been suggested as another technique for identifying a high testis.[13] Usually only minimal indications exist for performing these extensive studies because nearly all patients with true undescended testes require surgical exploration. It is imperative that a male with a nonpalpable testis undergo inguinal, retroperitoneal, and even intraabdominal surgical exploration, if necessary, to find the gonad or remnant, since malignant degeneration is particularly common in atrophic and/or intra-abdominal testes (see Chapter 13).

RETRACTILE TESTES

An extensive study of the human inguinal anatomy by Browne[14] in 1933 indicated that more than three fourths of testes not located in the scrotum of children were held in the higher position by an "overactive" cremaster muscle. These "retractile" testes have been termed pseudocryptorchid gonads[15] and are believed to behave in this manner because of an overactive cremasteric reflex combined with failure of complete attachment of the lower pole of the testis to the scrotum by the gubernaculum. By this normal muscular action, the testes are spontaneously held high during periods of stimulation, particularly when the thigh or abdomen is touched or when the boy is exposed to cold. Such testes may descend into the scrotum spontaneously when the child is asleep or relaxed, and when he is immersed in a warm bath. The spermatic vessels and vas deferens are of normal length in the retractile testis. Similarly, the morphologic features of retractile testes are normal compared to those in descended testes in boys of the same age.

Retractile testes usually are bilateral, although at least a third of the patients with this condition may have primarily unilateral involvement. During early adolescence the testis becomes larger than the external ring, the cremaster muscle becomes less active, and in most instances the retractile gonad remains in the scrotum thereafter. Browne[14] described a superficial inguinal pouch lying anterior to the external oblique fascia just superior to the external inguinal ring into which the retractile testis may ascend in many children (Fig 5-2). The roof of the pouch is formed by Scarpa's fascia and the posterior wall is formed by the external oblique aponeurosis. In many children with retractile testes, the gonad periodically ascends into the low inguinal canal through the external inguinal ring.

It is estimated that more than 50% of males with an empty scrotum who are younger than 11 years have retractile testes. In an extensive evaluation of more than 500 males of varying ages with retractile testes, Farrington[16] found that by the age of one year, 20% of testes were not visible in the scrotum on inspection; this figure rises to 25% and 30% at three and four years, respectively. After four years, the testis appears more frequently to be either definitely down, in a normal position, or up in the superficial inguinal pouch. An average of 9.8% of testes will be found in the latter position between four and 12 years of age, but beyond age 12, the testes can be expected to be in a normal position at the bottom of the scrotum (as were those of all the boys in the study[16]). In all of these patients, the gonads could be manipulated into a normal position in the scrotum at any age. Farrington[16] concluded that the peak of retractability is reached at five and six years, and from then onward there is a steady decrease in the number of testes that can be made to retract out of the scrotum with stimulation of the cremasteric reflex. At age 11, when 50% of boys show onset of puberty, about half of retractile testes can no longer be retracted out of the scrotum, and two years later it is rare for any testes to remain retractile.

Because a large percentage of boys with an empty scrotum have re-

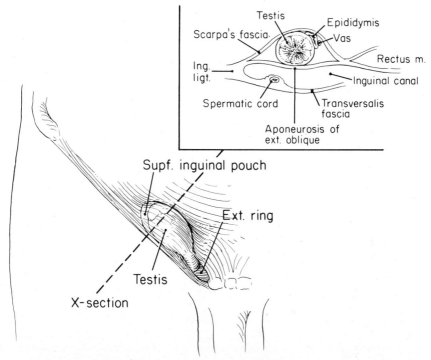

Fig 5–2.—Superficial inguinal pouch originally described by Browne[14] into which a retractile testis often ascends and in which a true cryptorchid testis frequently is located. Cross-section shows location of testis within pouch, bounded anteriorly by Scarpa's fascia and posteriorly by external oblique aponeurosis. Inguinal canal lies deep to external oblique layer and superficial to transversalis fascia. (From Fonkalsrud, E.W., *Curr. Probl. Surg.* 15:1, 1978. Used with permission.)

tractile testes that will descend spontaneously at puberty, it is important for the physician to distinguish between retractile and true undescended testes when he examines the patient. Lunderquist et al.[17] injected nitrous oxide intraperitoneally, looking for gas in the tunica vaginalis of true cryptorchid patients. Although transient administration of HCG will cause slight testicular enlargement and phallic growth, a short course may help to distinguish the retractile from the cryptorchid testis in those few patients in whom the testis cannot be manipulated into the scrotum. If descent into the scrotum occurs after a short one- to two-week course of about 10,000 units of HCG but the gonad subsequently retracts, therapy is not continued because there is no evidence that retractile testes will be improved either morphologically or functionally by permanent placement into the scrotum via hormone administration or by operation. Both spermatogenic and androgenic functions of retractile testes almost always are normal.

In a review of 43 adults who as children were diagnosed as having bilateral retractile testes, Puri and Nixon[18] found that the testicular volume was normal for age in each and that 74% of the married patients had children, a fertility rate similar to that for the normal adult population of the same age.

ECTOPIC TESTES

The true cryptorchid testis should be distinguished from an ectopic testis that has progressed normally through the inguinal canal and emerged from the external ring but that has been directed away from the scrotum into the thigh, suprapubic area, or perineum (Fig 5–3). Transverse ectopia to the contralateral groin has been reported.[19]

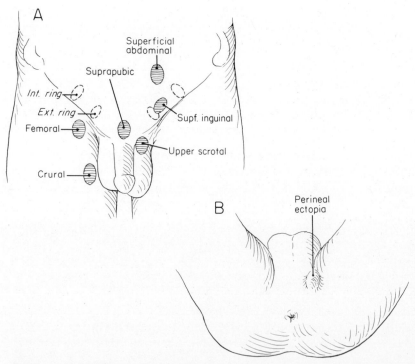

Fig 5–3.—A and **B,** typical locations for ectopic testes. Gonads in superficial inguinal pouch are considered truly undescended rather than ectopic. (From Fonkalsrud, E.W., *Curr. Probl. Surg.* 15:1, 1978. Used by permission.)

Jones[20] noted that more than 60% of operations for cryptorchidism in his hospital were performed for ectopia, although in almost all cases the gonads were found in the superficial inguinal pouch. For some years, it has been suggested that as high as 75% of ectopic testes are located in the superficial inguinal pouch; however, Scorer[21] and others have correctly indicated that these testes should be considered truly undescended rather than ectopic. In his review of 343 boys with undescended testes, Jones[20] classified ectopic testes as those diverging from the normal line of descent; this category included 248 of the patients, in only three of whom the gonad was positioned elsewhere than in the superficial inguinal pouch or behind the neck of the scrotum. The rarity of true ectopia is evidenced by the fact that in a review of more than 3,600 newborn males of whom 153 had testicular undescent, Scorer[21] found none with this anomaly. About 80% of reported ectopic testes are unilateral; they usually are normal in size, with normal spermatogenic and androgenic function. Regardless of location, they can be placed into the scrotum surgically because the spermatic cord is long enough to permit this procedure. Hormone therapy has no effect on movement of true ectopic testes into the scrotum.[20] Phillips and Holmes[22] reported torsion infarction involving interstitial ectopic testes in 17 spastic paraplegia patients and indicate that the condition may be difficult to differentiate from incarcerated inguinal hernia.

ANORCHISM

Normal male (wolffian) ductal development is dependent on fetal androgenic stimulation from the differentiated testis. With the complete absence of testicular tissue, female (müllerian) ductal development will differentiate into a feminine configuration. In rare instances, one testis may fail to develop (typically on the right), sometimes in association with ipsilateral agenesis of the kidney and ureter, in which case the anomaly has been termed the "right-sided syndrome."[23] The vas deferens in such patients usually is hypoplastic and ends blindly at the internal inguinal ring. The ipsilateral scrotum is likely to be undeveloped.

Anorchism was found to be unilateral in 27 and bilateral in six patients in a total of 988 operations performed for cryptorchidism by Gross and Jewett,[24] an incidence of 3.3%. Abeyaratne et al.[25] similarly found that 5.2% of 304 boys operated on for cryptorchidism had an absent testis, one fourth of which were bilateral. Jones[20] observed an identical figure of 5.2% with testicular hypoplasia or agenesis among

500 operations for undescended testis. The surgeon should be encouraged to seek a nonpalpable, high, undescended testis, inasmuch as total absence is uncommon.

Occasionally there is no evidence of viable testicular tissue on either side, although the external genitalia are fully differentiated in masculine configuration at birth and a vestigial vas deferens terminates blindly in the abdomen (Fig 5–4). Since these patients are both genotypic and fully masculinized phenotypic males, it is believed that the testis must have been present during early fetal development; hence, this condition of bilateral anorchism is often termed the "vanishing testis syndrome." Although the mechanism for the testicular absence is unknown, it may be secondary to torsion or to interference with blood supply during fetal development.[25] As the child grows, the penis remains small and nonpigmented, and the empty scrotum lies flat against the perineum. Puberty is delayed and characterized by persistent elevation of plasma FSH and LH levels and low plasma testosterone levels.

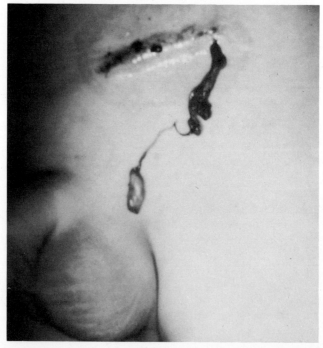

Fig 5–4.—Atrophic remnant of testis in four-year-old boy, showing excised spermatic cord and tiny vas extending to gonadal remnant. Prosthesis has been placed in scrotum. (From Fonkalsrud, E.W., *Curr. Probl. Surg.* 15:1, 1978. Used with permission.)

Conditions other than bilateral cryptorchidism can mimic anorchism. These include severe virilization of a female child caused by congenital adrenal hyperplasia or by maternal ingestion of certain hormones (androgens or some of the synthetic progestational agents) capable of virilizing the female fetus; idiopathic pseudohermaphroditism; true hermaphroditism; and the male counterpart of Turner's syndrome. The latter may be suggested by the finding of visceral and somatic anomalies usually observed in phenotypic females with Turner's syndrome. Thus early evaluation to distinguish bilateral anorchism from these conditions is essential to provide androgenic hormone replacement and to avoid the development of microgonadism and female body habitus.[26]

Rivarola et al.[27] recommend giving a course of HCG to males with bilateral nonpalpable testes to determine if anorchism is present. If high undescended testes are evident, the plasma testosterone level will increase significantly; however, if the patient is anorchidic, the testosterone level will not change. Although diagnostic ultrasound and the CAT scan may help to identify intra-abdominal testes, surgical exploration is necessary to establish the diagnosis. Exogenously administered testosterone therapy in early adolescence will produce a gratifying response of male sexual maturation. Testicular prostheses may be inserted into the scrotum at the time of exploration regardless of the patient's age; however, larger prostheses may be necessary after testosterone therapy has enlarged the scrotum.

REFERENCES

1. Hinman F. Jr.: Optimum time for orchidopexy in cryptorchidism. *Fertil. Steril.* 6:206, 1955.
2. Scorer C.G.: The descent of the testis. *Arch. Dis. Child.* 39:605, 1964.
3. Gross R.E.: *The Surgery of Infancy and Childhood. Its Principles and Techniques.* Philadelphia, W.B. Saunders Co., 1953.
4. Hamilton J.B., Hubert G.: Differential diagnosis of pseudocryptorchidism and true cryptorchidism. *Endocrinology* 21:644, 1937.
5. Gross R.E., Replogle R.L.: Treatment of the undescended testis; opinions gained from 1767 operations. *Postgrad. Med. J.* 34:266, 1963.
6. Rea C.E.: Further report on the treatment of the undescended testis by hormonal therapy at the University of Minnesota Hospitals; a discussion of spontaneous descent of the testis and an evaluation of endocrine therapy in cryptorchidism. *Surgery* 7:828, 1940.
7. Lattimer J.K., Smith A.M., Dougherty L.J., et al.: The optimum time to operate for cryptorchidism. *Pediatrics* 53:96, 1974.
8. Flinn R.A., King L.R.: Experiences with the midline transabdominal approach in orchiopexy. *Surg. Gynecol. Obstet.* 131:285, 1971.
9. Thompson W.O., Heckel N.J.: Undescended testes: Present status of glandular treatment. *J.A.M.A.* 112:397, 1939.
10. White J.J., Shaker I.J., Oh K.S.: Herniography: A diagnostic refinement in the management of cryptorchidism. *Ann. Surg.* 39:624, 1975.

11. Ben-Menachem Y., deBeradinis M.C., Jalinas R.: Localization of intra-abdominal testes by selective testicular arteriography: A case report. *J. Urol.* 112:493, 1974.
12. Amin M., Wheeler C.S.: Selective testicular venography in abdominal cryptorchidism. *J. Urol.* 115:760, 1976.
13. Czerniak P., Itelson J.: Spermatogenic activity test (S.A.T.) for evaluation of fertility in cryptorchidism. *Fertil. Steril.* 18:135, 1967.
14. Browne D.: Some anatomical points in operation for undescended testicle. *Lancet* 1:460, 1933.
15. Charney C.W., Wolgin W.: *Cryptorchidism.* New York, Hoeber Medical Division, Harper & Row, 1957.
16. Farrington G.H.: The position and retractability of the normal testis in childhood with reference to the diagnosis and treatment of cryptorchidism. *J. Pediatr. Surg.* 3:53, 1968.
17. Lunderquist A., Nommesen N., Rafstedt S.: Cryptorchidism. *Acta Paediatr. Scand.* 57:473, 1968.
18. Puri P., Nixon H.H.: Bilateral retractile testes — subsequent effects on fertility. *J. Pediatr. Surg.* 12:563, 1977.
19. Dajani A.M.: Transverse ectopia of the testis. *Br. J. Urol.* 41:80, 1969.
20. Jones P.G.: Undescended testes. *Aust. Paediatr. J.* 2:36, 1966.
21. Scorer C.G.: The descent of the testis. *Arch. Dis. Child.* 39:605, 1964.
22. Phillips N.B., Holmes T.W. Jr.: Torsion infarction in ectopic cryptorchidism: A rare entity occurring most commonly with spastic neuromuscular disease. *Surgery* 71:335, 1972.
23. Glenn J.F.: The prostate, seminal vesicles, penis, and testes, in Sabiston D.C. Jr. (ed.): *Davis-Christopher: Textbook of Surgery.* Philadelphia, W.B. Saunders Co., 1972, p. 1562.
24. Gross R.E., Jewett T.C. Jr.: Surgical experiences from 1222 operations for undescended testes. *J.A.M.A.* 160:634, 1956.
25. Abeyaratne M.R., Aherne W.A., Scott J.E.S.: The vanishing testis. *Lancet* 2:822, 1969.
26. Kolodny H.D., Kim S., Sherman L.: Anorchia: A variety of the "empty scrotum." *J.A.M.A.* 216:479, 1971.
27. Rivarola M.A., Bergada C., Cullen M.: HCG stimulation test in prepubertal boys with cryptorchidism in bilateral anorchia and in male pseudohermaphroditism. *J. Clin. Endocrinol. Metab.* 31:526, 1970.

6 / Comparison of the Morphology of Normal and Cryptorchid Testes

W. MENGEL, M.D.

K. WRONECKI, M.D.

F. A. ZIMMERMANN, M.D.

THE TERM CRYPTORCHIDISM encompasses several conditions that may have differing causes. Although the clinical classification includes abdominal testes, inguinal testes, and ectopic testes, this is merely a topical guideline and does not indicate why the testes failed to descend. The origins of these various types of testicular maldescent are complex; pathophysiologically there are at least three reasons for cryptorchidism:

1. Primary dysgenic: Various genetic defects are included in this group, e.g., Klinefelter's syndrome, the so-called male Turner syndrome, and the Moon-Bardet-Biedl syndrome. In the latter, the abnormal testes do not respond to stimulation by HCG. Moreover, primary damage occurring during intrauterine development leads to atrophy or even anorchism.

2. Endocrine: A lack of stimulation from maternal gonadotropin in the last two months of gestation during which testicular descent normally occurs may cause maldescent. Furthermore, an inborn error of testosterone synthesis in the fetus or pituitary disorders that reduce gonadotropin secretion may cause maldescent.

3. Anatomical: Peritoneal adhesions to the spermatic vessels, tight inguinal annulus, persistent opening in the umbilicus, or insufficient development of the gubernaculum can prevent the physiologic descent of the testis.

Investigations by several authors clearly indicate that the cryptorchid testis has a different morphological appearance from normal and also that there are severe pathologic changes that the normal testis from a male of the same age does not undergo. The testis that is correctly located shows special age-dependent morphological changes during the course of its development from infancy to adulthood. The pathomorphological changes of the cryptorchid testis, which can be clearly defined by electron microscopy, are caused by a congenital defect or by secondary alterations due to the malposition. No morphological criteria have been described that have accurately reflected subsequent clinical fertility of the gonad.

HISTORICAL REMARKS

Until recently, it was believed that the testis developed physiologically in certain defined phases, between which no notable changes occurred. In 1972 Staedtler and Hartmann[1] showed that the preadolescent testis underwent a slow linear growth between the first and 10th years of life, as evidenced by measurements of the weight of the testis, diameter of the seminiferous tubules, and number of spermatogonia. In 1977 Hadžiselimović[2] described similar findings and noted that the seminiferous tubular diameter increased continuously until the 12th year of life. During the 13th year, there is a sudden increase in the tubular diameter, and the formation of lumina becomes apparent.[3] The number of spermatogonia also increases markedly at this time.

Rising levels of testosterone production according to age were observed by Knorr,[4] Schollenberg et al.,[5] and Gupta and Butler.[6] An increase in plasma levels of FSH and LH was demonstrated by Midgley[7] and Odell et al.[8,9] as well as by Schalch and Bryson,[10] indicating a steady advance in testicular development.

DEVELOPMENT OF TESTICULAR STRUCTURES

The microscopic structure of the testis consists of seminiferous tubules with Sertoli cells and spermatogonia located within the tubules, peritubular connective tissue, and interstitial tissue in which the hormone-producing Leydig cells are located. The germinal epithelium develops during intrauterine growth; Hilscher[11] regards the development of the male gonadal cells as "early spermatogenesis." This stage is preceded ontogenically by the following two phases:

1. Pregonadal phase, at about the 20th week of gestation, when the primordial gonadal cells migrate from their first location in the vitelline sac to the primary gonadal field.

2. Prespermatogenic phase, at about the 35th week of gestation, when the testis develops from the undifferentiated gonad. The prospermatogonia arise from primordial gonadal cells called multiplying prospermatogonia, or M-prospermatogonia. Later, gonadal cells,

called transitional prospermatogonia, or T-prospermatogonia, are formed. For a considerable period these cells do not proliferate but later form the major portion of the gonadal cells in the developing seminiferous tubules.

In the full-term infant, A-spermatogonia develop from the T-prospermatogonia following birth. Histologically, two types of A-spermatogonia may be distinguished: the A-pale spermatogonia with a pale nucleus and the A-dark spermatogonia with a dark nucleus. The existence of a third type of spermatogonia cell, the so-called A-long type, has not been clearly defined. Furthermore, there are B-spermatogonia from which spermatocytes proliferate. The early spermatogenesis continues until puberty. Hadziselimović[2] discriminates the types further into fetal and transitional spermatogonia in addition to the A-pale and A-dark spermatogonia.

The Sertoli cells have different functions; they are believed to serve primarily as nutritive cells, are capable of phagocytosis, have supporting functions, and produce hormones as well. Vilar[12] and Hilscher[11] have identified only dark and pale Sertoli cells in the preadolescent testis. Hadžiselimović[2] has distinguished four types of Sertoli cells during gonadal development. The fetal Sertoli cells contain smooth and rough endoplasmic reticulum as well as lipids and lamellar bodies. The elliptic nucleus presents numerous invaginations. Following birth, the fetal Sertoli cell evolves into the SA-type of cell, the ultrastructure of which contains neither smooth endoplasmic reticulum nor lamellar bodies and is characterized by a round nucleus free of invaginations. In addition to SA-cells, SB types of Sertoli cells are present throughout childhood, located on the basement membrane; the nucleus is electron dense and has a rough surface with some invaginations. During the late prepubertal period, vacuoles and endoplasmic reticulum appear in the cytoplasm.

At the onset of puberty, the SA and SB cells change into SC cells, which increase in size sixfold compared with the fetal Sertoli cells, although they have a similar structure. In addition to nuclear invaginations, there are smooth as well as rough endoplasmic reticulum, numerous lipoid spots, and lamellar bodies. The wall of the seminiferous tubules consist of the basement membrane, on which the Sertoli cells and the spermatogonia are located, and the adjoining tunica propria. These structures are held together by elastic as well as collagenous fibers and by fibrocytes.

Although the Leydig cells are not altered in the cryptorchid testis, we wish to comment on their presence in the interstitial tissue. Vilar[12] indicates that the Leydig cells degenerate irreversibly within three months after birth, and that after three years no Leydig cells are present. According to Hatekeyama,[13] only a portion of the Leydig cells degenerate, whereas others undergo simple atrophy. These simple degenerated cells are demonstrable during the entire period of early childhood. Later, during puberty the adult Leydig cell is believed to develop from these atrophied cells. Hayashi and Harrison[14] demonstrated the presence of Leydig cells within the first year of life, and then again only after the fifth and sixth years. Hadžiselimović[2] identified Leydig cells during the first year of life; however, during the second and third years he found preliminary stages of Leydig cells in the interstitial tissues, which appeared to mature between the fourth and eighth years. Before puberty there is a second inactivity phase until the Leydig cells mature completely. Wronecki[15] was unable to demonstrate the presence of Leydig cells before the 10th year of life.

THE NORMALLY DESCENDED TESTIS

During the first two years of life, the seminiferous tubules are moderately tortuous with an epithelium consisting of two layers. Neither a strict morphological order nor lumina are present. The inner layer of the tubular wall is so thin that it can be detected only by electron microscopic photomicrographs. The tunica propria consists of a thin collagenous layer with fibroblasts; there are no elastic fibers. The spermatogonia reside on the basement membrane, and bright cytoplasm makes them easily detectable. Both fetal and T-spermatogonia are present, the former characterized by electron-light cytoplasm; a round nucleolus; and loose, thin-appearing chromatin, with a large centrally located nucleus. The mitochondria are concentrated around the nucleus. The T-spermatogonia are considerably smaller, with an oval nucleus consisting of delicate chromatin and a peripherally located nucleolus, and the mitochondria are located close to the nuclear membrane. The cytoplasm is denser than that in the fetal spermatogonia. Sertoli cells predominate during this period and are attached to the basement membrane by a narrow process. The cell membranes are somewhat meshed together, the cells containing more and larger mitochondria as well as more smooth endoplasmic reticulum than the spermatogonia. The oblong-shaped nuclei of the Sertoli cells show frequent invaginations, although several of the cells contain round nuclei. The cytoplasm contains free ribosomes, glycogen granules, and lipoid spots. In many instances the nuclei are located peripherally. The peritubular connective tissue, which functions as a border for the seminiferous tubules, is constructed from a delicate layer of tissue containing numerous fibroblasts.[16]

The interstitium during the first two years of life evolves into different patterns. The stroma may vary considerably in width, consisting of loose, partly reticular, and partly collagenous connective tissue containing numerous fibroblasts with blunt nuclei that are electron light. In addition, sparsely located fibrocytes with electron-dense, spindle-shaped nuclei are located between stretched collagenous fibers.

During the next two years, the morphological appearance of the testis remains much the same, although certain differences have been observed: the tubules are more tortuous and have a two-layered epithelium. The spermatogonia and Sertoli cells are identical in appearance, as they are during the first two years. The collagenous fibers within the tunica propria are more dense and the number of fibroblasts increases. The interstitial tissue appears loose and contains fibroblasts. The width of the interstitium may vary considerably. The fetal cell type of spermatogonia and Sertoli cells are no longer present.

Until the sixth year of life the seminiferous tubules become increasingly tortuous. Light microscopic studies show that the tubules are closely attached to each other, and the percentage of interstitial tissue decreases. The tubular epithelium develops three layers, although no lumen is present. The spermatogonia are easily distinguished from the Sertoli cells by their pale cytoplasm. The tunica propria appears as a narrow collagenous lamellar structure in the inner layer of the tubules. Only a few fibrocytes and fibroblasts are present in the peripheral layers. The interstitium is loose and contains fibrocytes and fibroblasts.

Between the sixth and 10th years of life, a marked increase in the diameter of the tubules becomes apparent and the epithelium clearly consists of three layers. There is no lumen or evidence to indicate the beginning of spermatogenesis. A delicate collagenous layer is present near the basement membrane. The tunica propria consists solely of fibrocytes. Spermatogonia and Sertoli cells similarly differ in their ultrastructure compared with the earlier stages. The interstitium consists primarily of fibroblasts.

After the 10th year of life, the tubular diameter increases noticeably. During the following years, the peritubular connective tissue increases in size, and the following morphological picture is observed: a broad layer of collagenous fibers is arranged longitudinally or circularly next to the basement membrane. Next to this layer is a cellular structure containing fibroblast-like cells that have centrally located nuclei with a membrane marked by several pores. The cytoplasm has long processes corresponding to tight junctions. There are many fibroblasts in the interstitium.

THE CRYPTORCHID TESTIS

The histologic appearance of the cryptorchid testis shows patho-logic differences from that described for the normal testis. By light microscopy the first changes can be noted during the third year of life, although they may be demonstrated much earlier by electron micros-copy. These morphological abnormalities are present in bilaterally undescended testes as well as in the unilaterally undescended testis. In patients with unilateral testicular undescent, morphological changes are also apparent in the contralateral scrotal-positioned testis, although these pathologic changes occur later.[17]

THE CRYPTORCHID TESTIS IN LIGHT MICROSCOPY

The seminiferous tubules of dystopic testes are lined with one or two layers of epithelium and contain immature precursors of Sertoli cells. A lumen is not present within the tubules. Measurements of the mean tubular diameter show normal values during the first two years of life; however, these values diminish beginning with the third year until puberty and are a definite sign of disturbed testicular develop-ment (Table 6–1).

Using a quantitative evaluation method,[18] it is clearly apparent that there is a statistically significant decrease in the number of spermato-gonia in undescended testes, which remains low throughout child-hood (Fig 6–1).[17] The basement membrane is delicate and shows an increase in width and fibrous tissue content.

The widening of the interstitium during the following years is caused by an increase in collagenous fibers. The stroma contains a greater quantity of fibrocytes and fibroblasts.

TABLE 6–1.—MEAN DIAMETER OF SEMINIFEROUS TUBULES CALCULATED FROM 20 MEASUREMENTS OF ONE SLIDE (INVESTIGATION OF 367 BIOPSIES OF CRYPTORCHID TESTES)

	MEAN DIAMETER OF TUBULES (μ)	
YR OF LIFE	Normal Range (Descended Testes)	Cryptorchid Testes
0–2	48–62	48–57
2.1–4	52–64	38–45
4.1–6	53–80	38–40
6.1–8	57–74	43–45
8.1–10	70	39–42
10.1–15	70–115	43–50

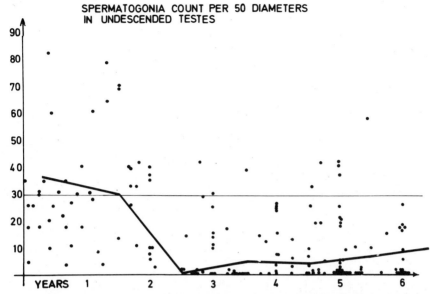

SPERMATOGONIA COUNT PER 50 DIAMETERS
IN UNDESCENDED TESTES

Fig 6–1. — Mean count of spermatogonia in undescended testes.

Leydig cells do not become visible before puberty. Electron microscopic studies of cryptorchid testes demonstrate pathologic changes on most testicular structures as early as the second year of life.[15, 19]

ULTRASTRUCTURE OF THE CRYPTORCHID TESTIS

During the first year of life there is no difference between a normal and cryptorchid testis as shown by electron microscopy. In the second year slight pathomorphological changes become evident, which gradually become more prominent, as shown in the following electron photomicrographs:

1. Spermatogonia. — Figure 6 – 2 shows the ultrastructure of a normal descended testis in a two-year-old boy. The big spermatogonia have a large, round nucleus and its nucleolus lies in an apical position. The nuclear membrane consists of two lamellar layers with numerous pores and does not show enlargement of the perinuclear space. The surrounding cytoplasm is less dense and contains a normal number of mitochondria with normal structures. The number of mitochondria may be greater in the spermatogonia and in the Sertoli cells. These mitochondria are elongated or round bodied; they are present in a condensed form and are shown on electron microscopy to have a less dense matrix (Fig 6 – 3). Smooth as well as granular endoplasmic retic-

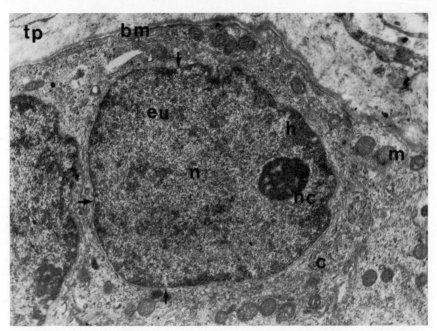

Fig 6–2. — Normally descended testis *(arrows)* in two-year-old patient; ×19,600. Spermatogonia attached to basement membrane without pathologic changes. *tp* = tunica propria; *bm* = basement membrane; *c* = cytoplasm; *n* = nucleus; *nc* = nucleolus; *m* = mitochondria; *h* = heterochromatin; *eu* = euchromatin.

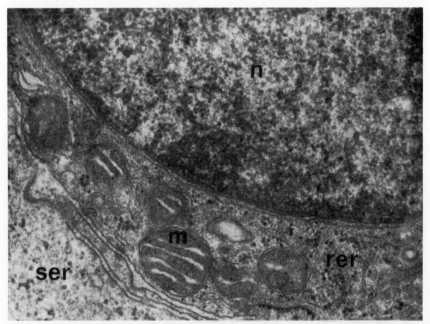

Fig 6–3. — Cryptorchid testis in eight-year-old patient; ×89,600. Mitochondria in cytoplasm in condensed form. *n* = nucleus; *m* = mitochondria, *rer* = rough endoplasmic reticulum; *ser* = smooth endoplasmic reticulum.

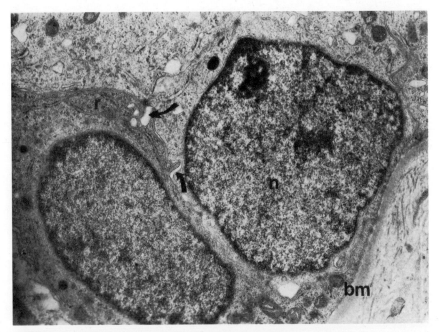

Fig 6–4. – Cryptorchid testis in six-year-old patient; ×22,400. Enlargement of intercellular space between two spermatogonia. *n* = nucleus; *r* = ribosomes; *bm* = basement membrane; *arrows* = intercellular space.

ulum, free ribosomes, and an enlargement of the intercellular space between the borders may be seen between two spermatogonia (Fig 6–4). The perinuclear space between the two layers of the nuclear membrane is enlarged. This phenomenon is present in spermatogonia (Fig 6–5) and also in the Sertoli cells (Fig 6–6).

The increase in number of mitochondria, decrease in number of ribosomes of the granular endoplasmic reticulum, and growing number of free ribosomes become evident primarily after the fifth year of life. By age nine, vacuolation of the cytoplasm occurs and vacuolar degeneration of the mitochondria becomes apparent. An increase in free ribosomes is a histologic characteristic of a cryptorchid testis at this age (Fig 6–7). The final status of a dystopic testis is shown in Figure 6–8 where a damaged but still demonstrable spermatogonium is present, and an autolyzed cell may be seen.

2. Sertoli Cells. – The Sertoli cells, which are smaller than the spermatogonia, are the supporting cells of the seminiferous tubules. Between the third and fifth years of life, there are many vacuoles and

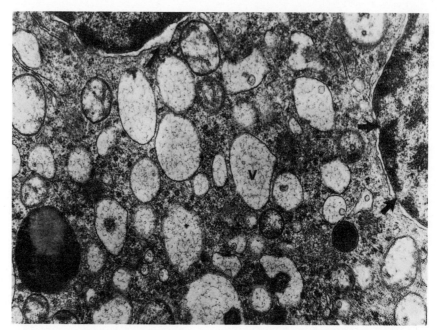

Fig 6–5.—Cryptorchid testis in two-year-old patient; ×33,600. Enlargement of perinuclear space and vacuolation of cytoplasm. *Arrows (at right)* = perinuclear space; *arrow (above left)* = pore of nuclear membrane; *v* = vacuole.

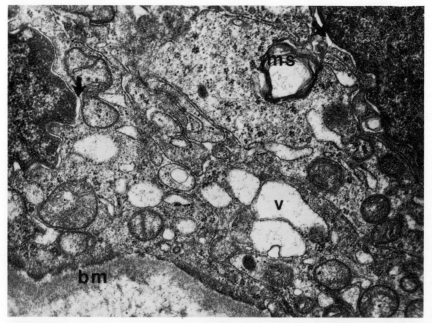

Fig 6–6.—Cryptorchid testis in 15-year-old patient; ×19,600. Sertoli cell with vacuolation of cytoplasm, deposition of myelin and enlargement of perinuclear space. *v* = vacuole; *bm* = basement membrane; *ms* = myelin structure; *arrow* = perinuclear space.

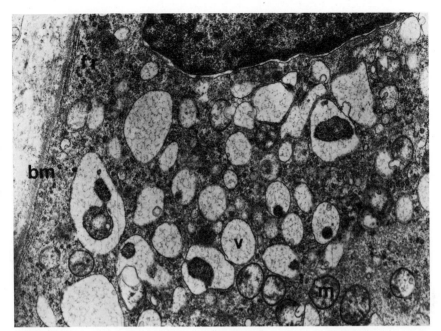

Fig 6–7.—Cryptorchid testis in 13-year-old patient; ×25,200. Vacuolic degeneration of cytoplasm and mitochondria of spermatogonia. *fr* = free ribosomes; *m* = mitochondria; *v* = vacuole; *bm* = basement membrane.

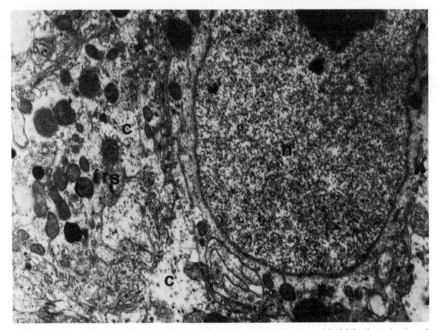

Fig. 6–8.—Cryptorchid testis in 13-year-old patient; ×25,200. Autolysis of spermatogonium (shown on left side). *n* = nucleus; *c* = cytoplasm; *frs* = fragments of spermatogonium.)

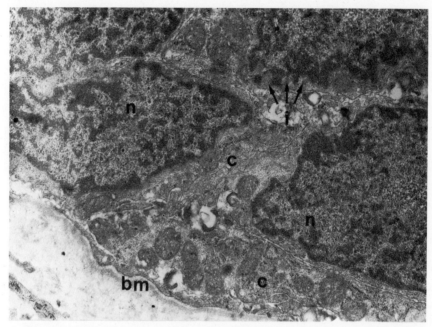

Fig 6–9.—Cryptorchid testis in two-year-old patient; ×25,200. Marked plication *(arrows)* of nuclear membrane *(i)* of Sertoli cell. *n* = nucleus; *c* = cytoplasm; *bm* = basement membrane.

numerous free ribosomes in the cytoplasm. The cytoplasm becomes fibrotic, and the nuclei have a heterogeneous chromatin pattern and a plicated nuclear membrane (Fig 6–9).

During subsequent years, the pathologic changes become more prominent, as seen in the cytoplasm of a damaged Sertoli cell (Fig 6–10). Fibrotic structures and fragments of the granular endoplasmic reticulum without ribosomes are present. The mitochondria are packed together, and in some cases there are no ribosomes in the cytoplasm. As with the spermatogonia, vacuolation of the intercellular spaces may occur, giving the appearance of empty bubbles (Fig 6–11).

During the prepubertal years, myelin may be deposited in the cytoplasmic vacuoles (see Fig 6–6); and lipofuscin deposits may be present (Fig 6–12).

3. Peritubular Connective Tissue.—Alterations in the morphological appearance of the peritubular connective tissue may be observed, depending on the age of the malpositioned testis. During the first year of life, the basement membrane is delicate and homogeneous, appear-

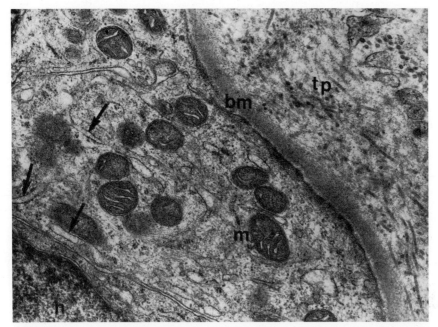

Fig 6–10.—Cryptorchid testis in six-year-old patient; ×39,200. Damaged Sertoli cell with fragments of rough endoplasmic reticulum without ribosomes. *n* = nucleus; *m* = mitochondria; *bm* = basement membrane; *tp* = tunica propria; *arrows* = rough endoplasmic reticulum without ribosomes.

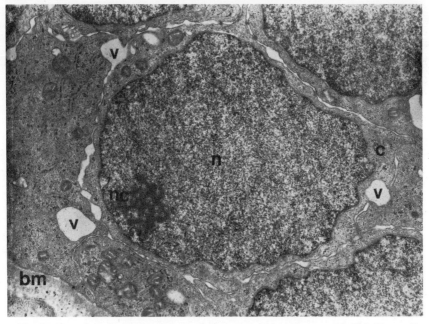

Fig 6–11.—Cryptorchid testis in eight-year-old patient; ×22,400. Vacuolic enlargement of intercellular spaces between two Sertoli cells. *n* = nucleus; *nc* = nucleolus; *c* = cytoplasm; *v* = vacuole; *bm* = basement membrane.

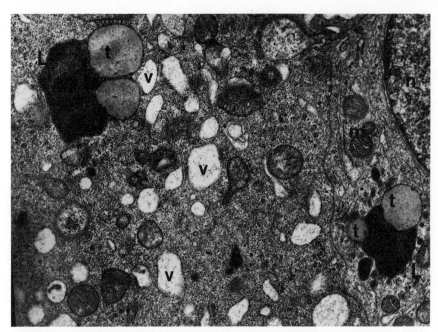

Fig 6–12.—Cryptorchid testis in 12-year-old patient; ×22,400. Fragments of Sertoli cells with vacuoles, fat, and lipofuscin deposits. *n* = nucleus; *v* = vacuole; *L* = lipofuscin; *t* = fat deposit; *m* = mitochondria.

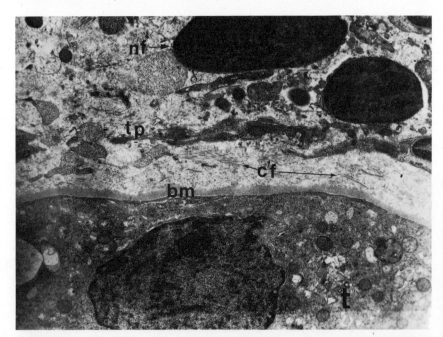

Fig 6–13.—Normally descended testis in two-year-old patient; ×14,000. Peritubular connective tissue. *t* = seminiferous tubule; *bm* = basement membrane; *tp* = tunica propria; *cf* = collagen fibers; *nf* = nucleus of fibroblast.

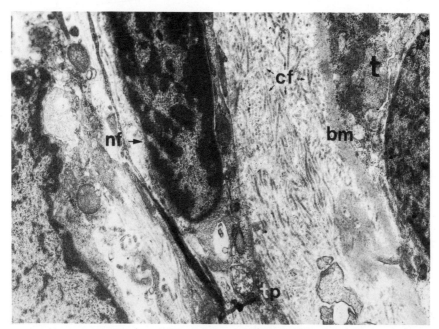

Fig 6–14.—Cryptorchid testis in two-year-old patient; ×22,400. Broadening and collagenization of peritubular connective tissue. *t* = seminiferous tubule; *bm* = basement membrane; *tp* = tunica propria; *cf* = collagen fibers; *nf* = nucleus of fibroblast.

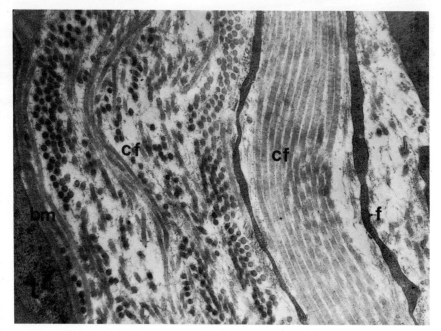

Fig 6–15.—Cryptorchid testis in 15-year-old patient; ×39,200. Bundled collagenic fibers oriented in different directions. *bm* = basement membrane; *cf* = collagen fibers; *f* = process of fibrocyte.

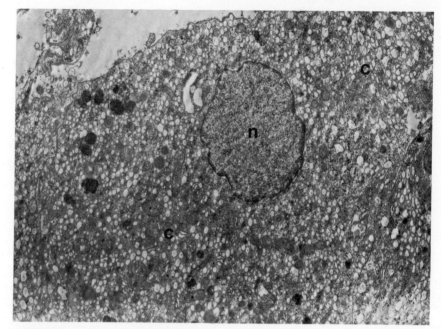

Fig 6–16. — Cryptorchid testis in 15-year-old patient; ×11,200. Undamaged Leydig cell. *c* = cytoplasm; *n* = nucleus.

ing similar to a normal testis (Fig 6–13). The tunica propria has only a few collagenous fibers. Over the following years, the tunica propria becomes thickened and the content of collagenous fibers increases. The direction of the collagenous fibers varies widely, as shown in Figure 6–14. Between the fifth and 10th years, the tunica propria enlarges markedly and the collagenous fibers become arranged in bundles oriented in different directions. Between these fibrous layers, narrow fibrocytes are occasionally apparent. Cell bodies located between two tubules may be seen in Figure 6–15.

4. Leydig Cells. — There are no apparent morphological changes in the Leydig cells compared to normal testes (Fig 6–16).

CONCLUSIONS

Morphological studies of cryptorchid testes do not show any pathologic changes other than malposition within the first 12 months of life. Beginning with the second year, histologic alterations become apparent on electron microscopic biopsy specimens. These changes are present in all structures of the parenchyma of the testis and become more abnormal as the malposition persists.

Light microscopic studies show a reduction of spermatogonia and an abnormal development of the seminiferous tubules, as demonstrated by the diminished diameters of the tubules and enlargement of the peritubular connective tissue. On electron microscopy the ultrastructure shows the following abnormal changes: there is a marked growth in the number of mitochondria, which later degenerate and develop vacuoles; the endoplasmic reticulum loses its ribosomes almost completely; the cytoplasm of the spermatogonia and the Sertoli cells may lose all ribosomes; an enlargement of the perinuclear space develops between the lamellae of the nuclear membrane in the Sertoli cells and the spermatogonia; the intercellular spaces are enlarged by numerous vacuoles.

The tunica propria is widened by a growing number of collagenous fibers, although the cause is not yet clear. Either primary pathologic changes of the spermatogonia in Sertoli cells, with secondary enlargement and collagenization of the peritubular connective tissue, or damage to the intratubular structures due to insufficient blood supply caused by a thickened and collagenous tunica propria may be factors.

Whether all of these changes in an undescended testis are owing primarily to congenital abnormalities, or are secondary to the abnormal position of the gonad cannot be answered from these studies. Clinical decisions can be made only on the basis of observations that the described pathomorphological changes (1) are absent during the first year of life in cryptorchid testes and (2) increase depending on duration of the malposition.

REFERENCES

1. Staedtler F., Hartmann R.: Histologische und morphometrische Untersuchungen zum praepuberalen Hodenwachstum bei normal entwickelten und zerebral geschädigten Knaben. *Dtsch. Med. Wochenschr.* 97:104, 1972.
2. Hadžiselimović F.: Cryptorchidism. Ultrastructure of normal and cryptorchid testis development. *Adv. Anat. Embryol. Cell Biol.* 53:3, 1977.
3. Seguchi H., Hadžiselimović F.: Ultramikroskopische Untersuchungen am Tubulus seminiferus bei Kindern von der Geburt bis zur Pubertät. I. Spermatogonienentwicklung. *Verh. Anat. Ges.* 68:133, 1974.
4. Knorr D.: Uber die Ausscheidung von freiem und glucuronsäuregebundenem Testosteron im Kindes- und Reifungsalter. *Acta Endocrinol. (Copenh.)* 54:215, 1967.
5. Schollenberg K., Seiler E., Hinkel G.K.: Die Ausscheidung von freiem und glucuronosidkonjugiertem Epitestosteron und Testosteron bei Kindern. *Z. Kinderheilkd.* 102:341, 1968.
6. Gupta D., Butler H.: Excretion of testosterone and epitestosterone glucuronid in preschool, preadolescent and adolescent children. *Steroids* 14:343, 1969.
7. Midgley A.R.: Radioimmunoassay for human follicle-stimulating hormone. *J. Clin. Endocrinol.* 27:295, 1967.

8. Odell W.D., Parlow A.T.: Radioimmunoassay for human follicle-stimulating hormone (HFSH). *Clin. Res.* 15:125, 1967.
9. Odell W.D., Ross G.T., Rayford P.L.: Radioimmunoassay for luteinizing hormone in human plasma or serum: Physiological studies. *J. Clin. Invest.* 46:248, 1967.
10. Schalch D.S., Bryson M.F.: Plasma luteinizing hormone levels in normal children and in subjects with pituitary and gonadal dysfunction: Determination by radioimmunoassay. *Pediatr. Res.* 1:308, 1967.
11. Hilscher W.: Beiträge der Spermatogenese des Menschen. Vortrag: Symposion "Prophylaktische Andrologie im Kindesalter." *Remscheid* 26:8, 1978.
12. Vilar O.: Histology of the human testis from neonatal to adolescence, in Rosenberg E., and Paulsen C.A. (eds.): *The Human Testis.* New York, Plenum Press, 1970, p. 95.
13. Hatekeyama S.: A study on the interstitial cells of the human testis, especially on their fine structural pathology. *Acta Pathol. Jpn.* 15:155, 1965.
14. Hayashi H., Harrison R.G.: The development of the interstitial tissue of the human testis. *Fertil. Steril.* 22:351, 1971.
15. Wronecki K.: Persönal communication, 1979.
16. Fawcett D.W., Leak L.V., Hedinger P.M.: Electron microscopic observations on the structural components of the blood-testis barrier. *J. Reprod. Fertil.* 10[suppl.]:105, 1970.
17. Mengel W., Hienz H.A., Sippell W.G., et al.: Studies on cryptorchidism: A comparison of histological findings in the germinative epithelium before and after the second year of life. *J. Pediatr. Surg.* 9:445, 1974.
18. Hedinger C.: Uber den Zeitpunkt frühest erkennbarer Hodenveränderungen beim Kryptorchismus des Kleinkindes. *Verh. Dtsch. Ges. Pathol.* 55:172, 1971.
19. Hadžiselimović F., Seguchi H.: Elektronenmikroskopische Untersuchungen beim Kryptorchismus. *Z. Kinderchir.* 12:376, 1973.

7 / Hormonal Influences on Testicular Development and Descent

F. HADŽISELIMOVIĆ, PH.D.
J. GIRARD, M.D.

DESCENSUS TESTIS is the process whereby the gonad moves from the dorsal wall of the abdomen into the scrotum. Since the beginning of this century, a disturbance of the hormonal control of this process has been regarded as the probable cause of cryptorchidism. In 1932 Engle[1] demonstrated in monkeys that premature descent of the testis occurred upon treatment with pregnancy urine or a water-soluble extract of the anterior pituitary. Rost[2] prevented testicular descent in experimental rodents by hypophysectomy. The introduction of hormonal treatment was the next logical step in the treatment of human cryptorchidism.[3] The success of gonadotropin therapy is believed to be attributable to the increased stimulation of androgen secretion.[4, 5] Androgen given alone also is often successful in treatment of cryptorchidism.[4, 6, 7] Finally, in human subjects the testes have been observed to descend in response to injection of androgens[6, 8] as in monkeys,[7] rats,[9] and ground squirrels.[10] Even if the testis is removed from the tunica albuginea in the newborn monkey and replaced by a paraffin ball, after which the tunica albuginea is reconstructed, testosterone administration causes descent of the paraffin testis into the scrotum.[11]

The experiments carried out with estradiol in gravid rodents remain unique today. Greene et al.[12] succeeded in producing cryptorchidism by treating gravid mice and rats with estradiol at the 13th day of gestation. Raynaud[13] repeated these experiments, proposing that cryptorchidism is the result of gubernacular atrophy, which in turn results from direct estradiol action on gubernacular growth. These experiments were important because of the opportunity to induce cryptorchidism without being forced to produce the condition by replacing already descended gonads in the abdomen.

Ontogenesis of the genital apparatus of the mouse repeats some phylogenic stages. At the 11th day of gestation, the gonads are situated in the urogenital anlage (Fig 7–1). The gonad at the 13th day is clearly distinguishable from the mesonephros and inguinal region, where it terminates in a small prominence. The gonads appear to be embedded in the entire length of the mesonephros. By the 15th day, the gubernaculum has become larger. The cranial pole derives from the mesonephros, and its caudal pole is attached by a funnel-shaped formation to the inguinal region. The cranial-caudal differentiation of the mesonephros develops further in a caudal direction. The ligamentum diaphragmale (LD) (which suspends the urogenital anlage in the embryonic mouse) is still present but is more elongated and leans against the dorsal abdominal wall. The transabdominal movement of the testis occurs as early as the 17th day of gestation when the gubernaculum changes in shape and is pushed against the lower abdominal wall. The caudal pole of the mesonephros has become somewhat smaller because the ductus deferens has separated from the mesonephros. The wolffian duct has more coils. At the 19th day of gestation, the gubernaculum is threadlike, inserting in the region of the future scrotum, an incudiform area, inverted in the abdominal cavity. The ligamentum diaphragmale is no longer recognizable.

Immediately after birth, the gubernaculum is recognized as a small, flat structure (see Fig 7–1). The epididymis is already formed and the processus vaginalis appears. The testis has terminated its transabdominal movement and now lies lateral to the bladder neck in the vicinity of the ventral abdominal wall. On the third postnatal day, the testis sinks into the processus vaginalis, and the ductus deferens and epididymis move in front of the gonad (see Fig 7–1). The actual scrotum is already developed. By the seventh postnatal day, the processus vaginalis has become deeper and wider; the cauda epididymis lies deep in the processus vaginalis and has more coils. Only remnants of the gubernaculum are visible. This is the period when the testis becomes larger. The caput epididymis is located at the level of the annulus inguinalis profundus. At the 14th day, the caudal scrotal tip is inverted and infolded. Between the scrotal tip and the cauda epididymis there is still a short connection, remnants of the gubernaculum. At the 21st

Fig 7–1.—Photomontage of testicular descent (DT) in the mouse, beginning on 11th day of gestation. *U* = urogenital anlage; *LD* = ligamentum diaphragmale. The course of DT is S shaped from dorsal-superior to ventral-inferior. Days of gestation number 13, 15, 17, and 19 as well as first, third,

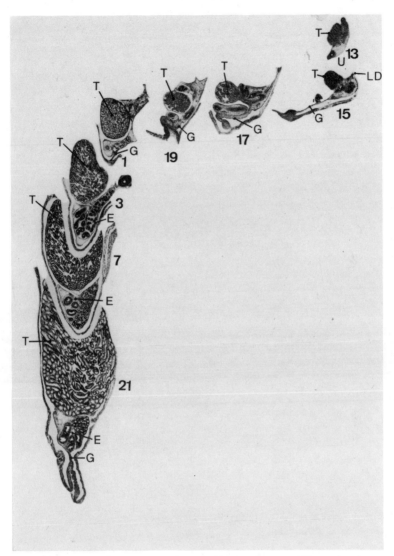

seventh, and 21st day after birth. Testis *(T)*, epididymis *(E)*, and gubernaculum *(G)* can be followed in their ontogenetic development. Magnification of all stages is the same, so that relative development of gonadal growth and cranio-caudal epididymis and ductus deferens differentiation is comparable. Note: gubernaculum never inserted directly into testis, and there is no extra-abdominal swelling of gubernaculum. The excessive testicular enlargement starts postnatally. (From unpublished dissertation by E. Kruslin, Basel Children's Hospital, Basel, Switzerland.)

postnatal day, the gubernaculum has attained its final form — a thread-like connection between scrotum and epididymis. The epididymis is fully developed and the testis lies in the scrotum.[14]

Estradiol (E_2B) administered at the 13th or 14th day of gestation leads to unilateral or bilateral cryptorchidism in 75–100% of all male newborn mice. Immediately after birth, in E_2B-cryptorchid mice, the testis remains in a dorsal position in contrast to the control mice, in which the testis is located between the ventral abdominal wall and bladder neck (Fig 7–2). In most animals treated with E_2B and HCG (70%), the testis is descended, as in the control mice (Fig 7–3). The position of the testes in the E_2B- and the E_2B plus HCG-treated animals was proportional to the degree of mesonephros development. The more the epididymis and ductus deferens were differentiated, the further the gonad had descended (see Fig 7–3). The appearance of

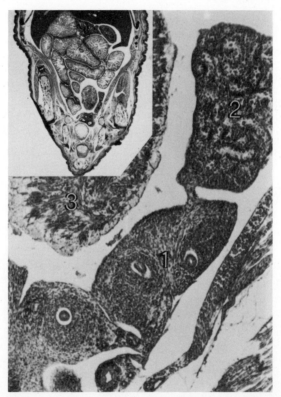

Fig 7–2. — Epididymis in one-day-old E_2B-treated mice: testis *(1)* lies posterior *(2)* to bladder *(3)*. Depletion of androgens causes differentiation of mesonephros stroma and inhibits development of wolffian duct.

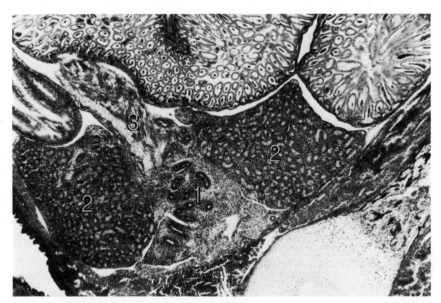

Fig 7–3. — Descended gonads in E₂B plus HCG-treated mouse. Sagittal section. Epididymis *(1)* is differentiated, showing more coils than in E₂B-treated mouse. Gonad *(2)*; bladder neck *(3)*.

the epididymis in E_2B-treated mice is completely different. The stroma, which consists of mesenchymal cells, is abundant and the cells are larger and polygonal. Generally they are less reduced in size and in degree of differentiation than in the control mice. The individual tubules of the epididymis are very few and have a multilayered epithelium (see Fig 7 – 2).[15] Although administration of estradiol hinders the transformation of the wolffian duct, this should not be regarded as a direct effect of estradiol on the mesonephros, but rather as the consequence of the androgen deficiency produced by insufficient stimulation of the Leydig cells by gonadotropins.[14] Simultaneous administration of HCG and E_2B prevents atrophy of the Leydig cells,[15] the wolffian duct becomes transformed into the vas deferens and epididymis, and descent takes place.[14]

There is thus strong evidence that intrauterine impairment of LH secretion and the consequent Leydig cell atrophy represent the main factor in the development of cryptorchidism. In connection with this concept, it is important to remember that the genetic findings in mutant mice with hypogonadism due to LH-RII deficiency suggest that the mutant is akin to Ever's series of human subjects with familial monotrophic pituitary insufficiency as an autosomal recessive LH-RH

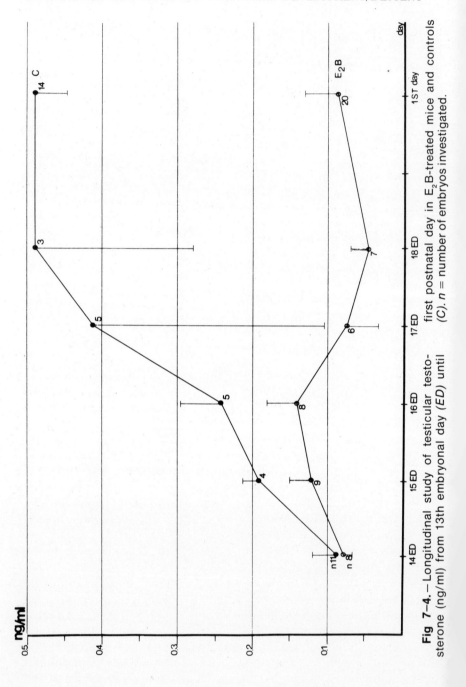

Fig 7–4.— Longitudinal study of testicular testosterone (ng/ml) from 13th embryonal day (ED) until first postnatal day in E_2B-treated mice and controls (C). n = number of embryos investigated.

TABLE 7-1.— TESTICULAR TESTOSTERONE CONTENT
IN ADULT MICE

ADULT MALE MICE	NO. OF TESTES EVALUATED	SERUM TESTOSTERONE (ng/ml) X	TESTOSTERONE (ng/testis) sd
E_2B-treated	22	0.07	0.11
Controls	12	0.53	0.46

deficiency. These mice are cryptorchid and sterile.[16] Moreover, in connection with hormone-dependent descent, there also is an absence of androgen-dependent differentiation of male genitalia as well as organ insensitivity to androgen in testicular feminization of the mouse. Affected mice have male genotypes, female phenotypes, and cryptorchid testes.[17] Parallel to the ultrastructural appearance of the Leydig cells in cryptorchid E_2B mice, which is atrophic, there also is a low testicular testosterone content (Fig 7-4). In such cryptorchid mice the testicular testosterone content remains lower even in adulthood.[18]

In spontaneously cryptorchid mice, the testicular testosterone content also is lower than in adult controls of the same age (Table 7-1). Similarly, a reduced testicular testosterone content is observed in congenitally cryptorchid pigs[19] and dogs.[20]

If LH-RH insufficiency is postulated to be a main factor in the cause of cryptorchidism, it seems logical that treatment with LH-RH would be successful. For this purpose, we performed an experimental study in spontaneously cryptorchid mice. When these mice are treated with 5 μg of LH-RH daily, results in 90% of cases are successful (11 of 12 testes descended after two weeks' therapy). The mean testicular testosterone value, which in cryptorchid mice is 6.2 ± 6.3 ng/ml, increases after two weeks of treatment in all mice to >21.5 ng/ml (control 15.5 ± 4.9 ng/ml).

CLINICAL OBSERVATIONS

Several clinical observations indicate a connection between gonadotropin insufficiency and cryptorchidism. In Kalman's syndrome, which is characterized by congenital aplasia or hypoplasia of the pituitary gland and anencephaly, the testes frequently are undescended. All cryptorchid boys in our study had atrophy of the Leydig cells as early as the first two weeks after birth (Figs 7-5 and 7-6). This atrophy is observed throughout childhood and is due to impaired

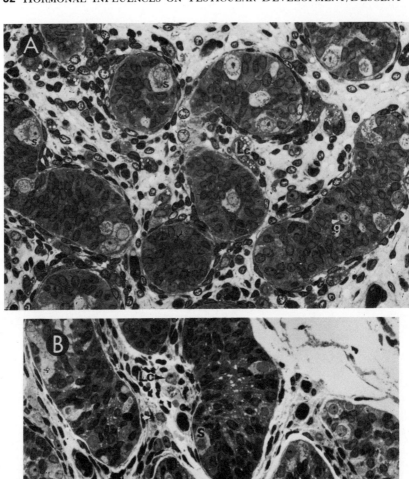

Fig 7–5.—A, semi-thin sections from two-week-old infant with normal descended testis, showing developed Leydig cells *(Lc) (arrowheads)*. Tubuli seminiferi contain gonocytes *(g)* and fetal spermatogonia *(S)*; ×20. **B,** two-week-old cryptorchid testis, which, in contrast, has only a few atrophic Leydig cells *(Lc)*. Tubulus seminiferus predominantly contains Sertoli cells, but fetal spermatogonia *(S)* and occasional gonocytes *(g)* are visible; ×20.

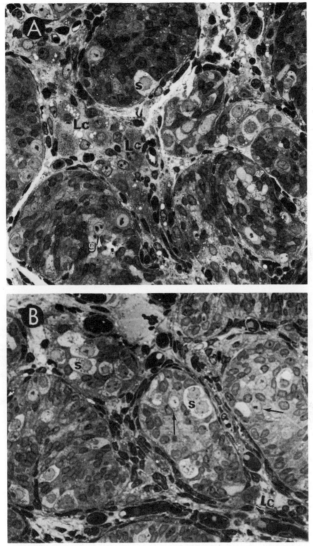

Fig 7–6. — **A,** five-week-old normally descended testis. Interstitium is full of enlarged Leydig cells *(Lc),* a sign of increased stimulation. Tubuli semini-feri contain gonocytes *(g)* and spermatogonia *(s)* in addition to Sertoli cells; ×20. **B,** five-week-old cryptorchid testis. Note that there is no physiologic increase in size and number of Leydig cells. Atrophic Leydig cells *(Lc)* are still visible. Gonocyte indicated by *arrows; s* = fetal spermatogonium; ×20.

stimulation[18, 21] rather than to a congenital malformation of the Leydig cells[22] or to secondary damage.[23]

Plasma testosterone levels are lower in cryptorchid infants than in infants with physiologically delayed descent or normal testicular descent.[24] Diminished plasma testosterone content also has been reported in cryptorchid adults.[25] It must be stated, however, that most investigators have found normal plasma testosterone levels in childhood, and almost all cryptorchid boys have a normal puberty. It is clear, therefore, that the underlying defect must be incomplete. Growth and bone age of cryptorchid boys likewise do not differ from those in the normal population, which in turn supports the theory that the gonadotropin deficiency is an isolated one.

In research into cryptorchidism, particular attention has always been paid to the germ cells as the most important criterion of quality of the tissue. However, there is still controversy about the cause of spermatogonia damage. Some investigators[26, 27] interpret the lack of spermatogonia, in some cases at least, as due not to any secondary dis-

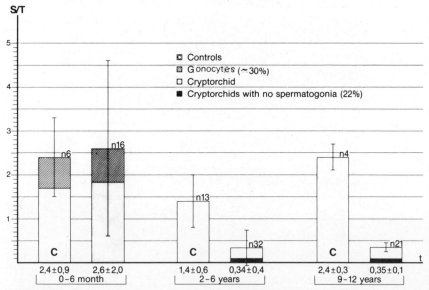

Fig 7–7.—Spermatogonia count per tubule (S/T) as related to age in controls *(C)* and cryptorchid boys (50 tubules per biopsy counted). Note that, particularly within first three months of life, there are about 30% gonocytes and 70% spermatogonia. In this case the transient forms between gonocyte and spermatogonium were counted as spermatogonia. After age two years, the S/T count is less than one-third that of normal controls; this difference in S/T count becomes even more pronounced after age nine.

turbance, but to a congential malformation. However, it seems important here to stress that within the first six months of life there is no lack of spermatogonia in cryptorchid testes (Fig 7–7). Furthermore, there is no significant difference in the spermatogonia count of cryptorchid and control testes. By deducting the number of gonocytes from the total number of germ cells, it becomes clear that there is no "physiologic decrease" in the number of spermatogonia in the first year of life, as seen by Koch et al.[28] and Hedinger.[27] On the other hand, there is a marked decrease in the number of spermatogonia per tubule in cryptorchid boys after the age of two years compared to boys with normally descended testes.

Among the cryptorchid boys in P_1 stage of puberty, according to Tanner, the mean plasma values for LH are basal 3.6 ± 2.2 IU/L and peak 7.7 ± 5 IU/L; for FSH: basal 1.85 ± 1.7 IU/L and peak 5.2 ± 3.3 IU/L; and for testosterone: basal 0.42 ± 0.1 ng/ml—all in the normal range.[29]

If histopathologic findings are taken as the parameter, the group with no spermatogonia can be recognized in the second, and particularly in the third, year of life. Compared with the group in which the number of spermatogonia per tubule (S/T) is only moderately reduced (S/T ≥ 0.5), there is a considerable difference in both LH and FSH values (Fig 7–8, and Table 7–2). However, a group with S/T = 0 is already recognizable within the first six months of life. The mean number of spermatogonia during that period in cryptorchid boys is the same as in the controls, but about 20% of cryptorchids already evidence a low spermatogonia count (S/T = 0.2–0.8). This group loses germ cells completely as early as the second year, and particularly in the third year of life. The ratio of 20% without spermatogonia to 80% with a reduced number of spermatogonia remains the same until puberty.

These studies indicate that there is a crucial point with regard to the optimal time for therapy for cryptorchidism. If we postulate that there is a physiologic increase in maturation after the testis is brought down,[22] even in cryptorchid boys with a hypogonadotropic axis, there is still a chance of fertility, providing the testis is brought into the proper position by hormonal or surgical means within the first or at the beginning of the second year of life. The first reports reviewing clinical experience with this concept of treatment[30] showed that over 90% of all cryptorchid boys operated on within the first two years of life are completely fertile in adulthood. These optimistic results may apply to 80% of cryptorchid boys. However, further investigation is necessary to ascertain whether patients with marked insufficiency of the pitu-

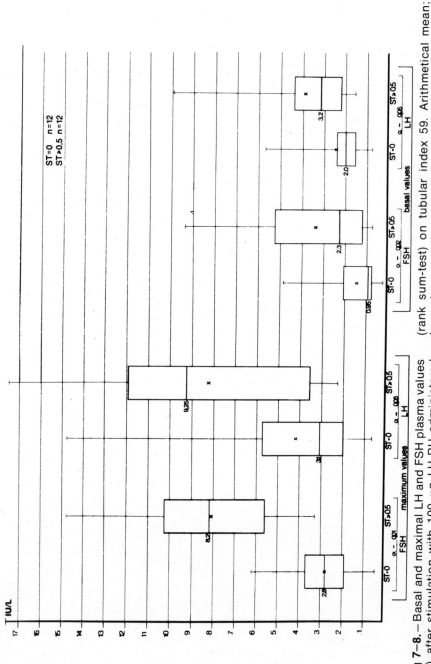

Fig 7–8.— Basal and maximal LH and FSH plasma values (IU/L) after stimulation with 100 μg LH-RH administered intravenously in 12 cryptorchid boys with S/T ratio = 0 and in 12 cryptorchid boys with S/T > 0.5. Wilcoxon test (rank sum-test) on tubular index 59. Arithmetical mean; *bar* = interquartile range; *line* drawn within bars = median and range.

TABLE 7–2.—BASAL VALUES FOR LH AND FSH FROM EIGHT CONTROLS AND 53 CRYPTORCHID BOYS (P_1 STAGE OF PUBERTY ACCORDING TO TANNER)

	S/T CONTROL ⩾2	S/T = 0	S/T >0 <0.5	S/T ⩾0.5
LH (mIU/ml)	4.3 ± 2.2	2.5 ± 2.2	3.9 ± 1.9	4.0 ± 2.7
FSH (mIU/ml)	1.3 ± 0.7	1.5 ± 1.3	1.36 ± 0.89	3.4 ± 2.9
No. of patients and % of distribution	8 (100%)	12 (22%)	29 (56%)	12 (22%)

S/T = spermatogonia per tubule.

itary-gonadal axis require substitution therapy to achieve full fertility. A direct relationship between LH function and the number of spermatogonia is strongly suggested by both the reduced number of spermatogonia in low LH responders and the low LH response in boys with no spermatogonia. This suggests a connection between testicular descent, the development of spermatogonia, testicular endocrine function, and gonadotropins, particularly LH.

Basal FSH values are higher in the group in which S/T ≥ 0.5, than in the control group and other cryptorchid groups in which S/T < 0.5 (see Table 7–2). The increased FSH in cryptorchid boys may be interpreted as a cause of germinal cell deficiency[31] or as a sensitive feedback mechanism between the pituitary release of FSH and the number of spermatogonia.[32] The increase in FSH appears to be the factor causing the higher number of germ cells in cryptorchid boys in the group in which S/T ≥ 0.5, despite the fact that they are of the same age and that gonadal position is similar to that in the group in which S/T = 0. Since the basal FSH value in this group (S/T = 0) is considerably lower than in the group in which S/T ≥ 0.5, it may be assumed that in the group in which S/T = 0, as well as in the group in which the S/T > 0 and < 0.5, no compensatory FSH excretion occurs as a result of hypophyseal insufficiency.

Although LH-RH therapy for cryptorchidism was introduced in 1975, its effectiveness is still controversial. The main criticism, which also applies to HCG treatment, is that testes that descend following this therapy are retractile, with normal histologic features and fertility potential and thus are not truly cryptorchid. A randomized clinical study using LH-RH therapy was devised as a means of resolving this controversy; the results are summarized as follows: 31 of 62 cryptorchid patients aged two to six years were randomly selected and surgically repaired immediately, biopsy specimens being obtained for light and electron microscopy. The remaining 31 patients received 1.2 mg of LH-RH nasal spray daily for four weeks. All the boys diagnosed as cryptorchid were examined independently by two pediatric surgeons.[33]

In 16 of 31 patients treated with LH-RH, testicular descent had occurred by the end of treatment. Fifteen patients treated unsuccessfully were operated on within two weeks after cessation of therapy, and biopsies done. In the group undergoing orchiopexy (no hormonal treatment), all biopsies showed typical signs of cryptorchidism, i.e., reduced number of spermatogonia, atrophy of Leydig cells, and thickening of peritubular tissue. The main histologic and ultrastructural differences compared with those in untreated patients were evident in the appearance of the Leydig cells, whereas the tubule diameter, histologic appearance of the spermatogonia, and number of spermatogonia remained unchanged. The LH-RH–treated group had an S/T of 0.31 ± 0.5 compared to 0.35 ± 0.5 in untreated controls. The most striking feature of the Leydig cells after LH-RH treatment is the marked increase in cell size and smooth endoplasmic reticulum.[34] These changes are identical to those observed after HCG treatment. Apart from the stimulatory signs, there also is an increase in recruitment of precursor Leydig cells from fibroblasts.

These results are in contrast to those observed for cryptorchid adults with gonadal damage, in whom extremely high LH and FSH values are the rule. It may be conjectured from this that primary LH and FSH insufficiency disappears during puberty, whereas the morphologically determinable damage to the testes arising from this deficiency is irreversible.

All boys treated with LH-RH underwent a short LH-RH stimulation test at the conclusion of therapy (100 μg LH-RH given intravenously). The maximal LH levels were measured after 30 minutes. Whereas the basal LH values did not differ between the groups in which treatment was successful or unsuccessful, the maximum values in the group showing no descent were noticeably lower, although still capable of stimulation. Since these cryptorchid boys represented a random selection from a defined basic group, we may conclude that successful treatment in cryptorchid boys depends on repeated high-peak LH secretions (Table 7–3).

Treatment with HCG of an amount totaling less than 10,000 IU does not yield as favorable results as high doses,[35] but the latter could be potentially hazardous. The choice, therefore, remains difficult. Human chorionic gonadotropin treatment is successful in about 30% of all cases.[35] In view of the objections to HCG treatment and the 50% success rate for LH-RH therapy, as well as the mode of application,

TABLE 7–3.— Basal and Peak LH Plasma Values (IU/L) in Successfully and Unsuccessfully Treated Cryptorchid Boys (2–6 Years of Age) After Four Weeks of LH-RH Therapy (1.2 mg/day)

NO. OF PTS.	BASAL VALUES		PEAK VALUES	
	SUCCESS	NO SUCCESS	SUCCESS	NO SUCCESS
1	4.6	3.6	15.8	2.8
2	4.2	0.8	10.4	4.6
3	0.8	3.2	14.6	8.2
4	0.8	0.8	11.2	2.7
5	3.1	3.0	7.0	14.8
6	6.0	4.6	9.6	5.8
7	2.0	2.3	6.4	4.8
8	4.0	0.8	8.0	5.4
9	4.6	4.2	9.4	2.6
10	1.2	2.0	6.8	2.0
11	1.8	1.4	5.8	4.4
Median	3.1	2.3	9.4°	4.6°

°2 α <0.01 Wilcoxon rank sum-test.

LH-RH treatment is to be preferred. Only patients who have inguinal hernia and painful cryptorchid testes require immediate surgery. We prefer to treat patients between the ninth and 12th months of life with hormone stimulation. If descent does not occur, we recommend performing an orchiopexy early in the second year of life.

REFERENCES

1. Engle E.T.: Experimentally induced descent of the testis in the Macacus monkey by hormones from the anterior pituitary and pregnancy urine. *Endocrinology* 16:513, 1932.
2. Rost F.: Versuche zum Descensus testiculorum. *Langenbecks Arch. Chir.* 177:680, 1933.
3. Schapiro B.: Ist der kryptorchismus hormonell oder chirurgisch zu behandeln? *Dtsch. Med. Wochenschr.* 38:38, 1931.
4. Wells L.J.: Descent of the testis. *Surgery* 14:436, 1943.
5. Backhouse K.M.: The gubernaculum testis hunteri: Testicular descent and maldescent. *Ann. R. Coll. Surg. Engl.* 35:15, 1964.
6. Hamilton J.B.: The effect of male hormone upon the descent of the testis. *Anat. Rec.* 70:533, 1938.
7. Hamilton J.B.: Therapeutics of testicular dysfunction. *J.A.M.A.* 116:1903, 1941.
8. Thompson W.O., Hackel N.J.: Undescended testes: Present status of glandular treatment. *J.A.M.A.* 112:397, 1939.
9. Reifer J., Walsh C.P.: Hormonal regulation of testicular descent: Experimental and clinical observations. *J. Urol.* 118:985, 1978.
10. Wells L.J., Overholser M.D.: Sperm formation induced by androgens following anterior pituitary removal. *Anat. Rec.* 73[suppl. 2]:56, 1939.

11. Martins T.: La testostérone peut provoquer la descente de testicules artificiels de paraffine. *C. R. Soc. Biol.* 131:299, 1938.
12. Greene R.R., Burill M.W., Ivy A.C.: Experimental intersexuality. The production of feminized male rats by antenatal treatment with estrogens. *Science* 88:130, 1938.
13. Raynaud A.: Modification expérimentale de la différentiation sexuelle des embryons des souris par action des hormones androgènes et oestrogènes. Paris, Herman et Cie, 1942.
14. Hadžiselimović F., Herzog B., Kruslin E.: Estrogen induced cryptorchidism in animals, in Hafez E.S.E., Nijhoff M. (eds.): *Descended and Cryptorchid Testis, Clinics of Andrology.* The Hague, in press.
15. Hadžiselimović F., Herzog B., Kruslin E.: The morphological background of estrogen-induced cryptorchidism in the mouse. *Fol. Anat. Jugos.* 8:63, 1978.
16. Cattanach B.M.: Gonadotrophin-releasing hormone deficiency in a mutant mouse with hypogonadism. *Nature* 269:338, 1977.
17. Blackburn W.R., Kying W.C., Bullock L., et al.: Testicular feminization in the mouse. Studies of the Leydig cell structure and function. *Biol. Reprod.* 9:9, 1973.
18. Hadžiselimović F., Girard J.: Pathogenesis of cryptorchidism. *Hormone Res.* 8:76, 1977.
19. Hanes F.M., Hooker C.W.: Hormone production in undescended testis. *Proc. Soc. Exp. Biol. Med.* 35:549, 1937.
20. Eik-Nes K.B.: Secretion of testosterone by the eutopic and the cryptorchid testis in the same dog. *Can. J. Physiol. Pharmacol.* 44:629, 1966.
21. Hadžiselimović F., and Herzog B.: The meaning of the Leydig cell in relation to the etiology of cryptorchidism. *J. Pediatr. Surg.* 11:1, 1976.
22. Kleinteich B.: Klinische Problematik, in Kleinteich B., Hadžiselimović F., Hesse V., et al. (eds.): *Kongenitale Hodendystopien. Modern Pädiatrie.* Leipzig, Georg Thieme Verlag, 1979.
23. van Straaten H.W.M., Ribbers-de Ridder R., Wensing C.J.G.: Early deviations of testicular Leydig cells in the naturally unilateral cryptorchid pig. *Biol. Reprod.* 19:171, 1978.
24. Gendrel D., Job J.C., Roger M.: Reduced postnatal rise of testosterone in plasma of cryptorchid infants. *Acta Endocrinol. (Copenh.)* 89:372, 1978.
25. Raboch J., Starka L.: Plasmatic testosterone in bilateral cryptorchids in adult age. *Andrology* 4:107, 1972.
26. Farrington G.H.: Germinal cell deficiency of the undescended testis: A congenital defect. *Surg. Forum* 20:540, 1969.
27. Hedinger C.: Histological data in cryptorchidism, in Job J.C. (ed.): *Cryptorchidism Diagnosis and Treatment.* Basel-Munich-Paris-London-New York-Sydney, S. Karger, 1979.
28. Koch H., Rahlf G., Mühlen A., et al.: Endokrinologische und morphologische Untersuchungen beim Maldescensus Testis. *Dtsch. Med. Wochenschr.* 100:683, 1975.
29. Hadžiselimović F., Girard J., Herzog B.: Treatment of cryptorchidism by synthetic luteinizing-hormone-releasing hormone. *Lancet* 2:1125, 1977.
30. Ludwig G., Potempa J.: Der optimale Zeitpunkt der Behandlung des Kryptorchidismus. *Dtsch. Med. Wochenschr.* 100:680, 1975.

31. Waaler P.E.: Endocrinological studies in undescended testes. *Acta Pae-diatr. Scand.* 65:559, 1976.
32. Sizonenko P.C., Schindler A.M., Roland W., et al.: FSH III. Evidence for a possible prepubertal regulation of its secretion by the seminiferous tubules in cryptorchid boys. *J. Clin. Endocrinol. Metab.* 46:301, 1978.
33. Hoecht B.: Personal communication.
34. Hadžiselimović F., Baumann J., Girard J.: Ultrastructure of the cryptorchid Leydig cells after LH-RH treatment. *Acta Endocrinol. (Copenh.)* [suppl.] vol 225, 1979.
35. Canlorbe P., Laclyde J.P., Toublanc J.E., et al.: Results of treatment with human chorionic gonadotropin in cryptorchidism, in Job J.C. (ed.): *Cryptorchidism: Diagnosis and Treatment.* Basel-Munich-Paris-London-New York-Sydney, S. Karger, 1979.

8 / Androgenic Function of the Cryptorchid Testis

BARBARA LIPPE, M.D.

THE TESTIS INITIATES its androgenic role in the fetus while still in the original embryologic intra-abdominal site. The gonadal primordium begins testicular differentiation at the 15- to 17-mm stage with the appearance of seminiferous tubules, followed by the development of interstitial cells at the 28- to 30-mm stage. In a series of experiments, Jost[1] demonstrated that subsequent organization of the mesonephric (wolffian) duct into the masculine structures, including epididymis, vas deferens, and seminal vesicles, is dependent on the local secretion of testicular testosterone. These events, occurring at the 30- to 60-mm stage, are thus the result of an active androgenic secretion of the fetal testis. The effect can be blocked by antiandrogen and mimicked by locally placed testosterone crystals.

This embryologic differentiation occurs independently on each side of the fetus. No local diffusion of testosterone from one genital ridge appears to influence the events on the contralateral side. The postnatal presence of paired sex accessory structures therefore implies that functional testicular tissue was present prenatally whether it is subsequently demonstrated or not. Similarly the developing testicular Sertoli cell secretes a nonsteroidal locally active substance,[2, 3] which causes müllerian regression in a bilateral fashion at about the same stage (30–60 mm). Again, contralateral diffusion of this so-called müllerian inhibiting substance or anti-müllerian hormone does not appear to occur, and so the absence of müllerian structures in combination with an atrophic or absent testis suggests early fetal activity for the gonad.

Finally, androgenic secretion of the intra-abdominal fetal testis is responsible for the virilization of the external genitalia of the male.[4] Testosterone is secreted into the fetal circulation to reach its target tissues. In the case of the genital tubercle, prepuce, and genital folds, the testosterone is converted locally by tissue 5 α-reductase to DHT and it is the DHT that causes virilization. The process of elongation of the tubercle and fusion of the median raphe begins at about the 40-mm stage (65–70 days) and reaches the stage of physiologic hypospadias by 70 mm (90–100 days).[5] The concentration of testosterone required for complete external virilization is not known, although the fetal serum levels reached at this time are in the range of the pubertal male.[6] Cryptorchid males usually do not have defects in virilization, again implying adequate testicular function in utero.

In the neonate the testis is still hormonally active. Studies of testosterone secretion in the first year of life demonstrate a brisk rise in testosterone to midpubertal levels in the first one to two months followed by a subsequent fall to prepubertal values by six to 12 months.[7] The physiologic significance of this early testosterone surge is unknown. In infants with cryptorchidism, unilateral or bilateral, longitudinal studies of testosterone secretion in the first year have not been published. However, cross-sectional studies include patients with cryptorchidism and suggest that this early surge occurs.[8]

Between the nadir of the neonatal testosterone surge and the onset of puberty, gonadal steroid secretion normally is low. There are no apparent differences between plasma testosterone concentrations in males and females prior to age 12 or until puberty is well underway in the male.[9, 10] In cryptorchid males, basal plasma testosterone concentrations are reported to be the same as normal[11] or lower, and basal urinary testosterone excretion is variously reported as being normal, lower, or higher.[12] Consequently, the question of actual integrated testosterone secretion during this period in the cryptorchid male is unclear. However, the functional significance of the potentially small differences that may exist in some patients during the prepubertal years seems to be minimal. Abnormalities in prepubertal somatic growth or development have not been noted in otherwise normal cryptorchid males. Moreover, in a series of patients subsequently demonstrated to be anorchidic, prepubertal growth was normal, and no eunuchoid upper:lower body segment ratios were seen.[13] Thus there is no evidence that cryptorchidism or anorchism results in a clinically deficient androgenic state prior to puberty.

Studies designed to evaluate the hypothalamic-pituitary-testicular axis in cryptorchidism, however, have demonstrated abnormalities in feedback control even in prepubertal patients. In the prepubertal male, testosterone is the major feedback regulator of LH secretion, whereas a nonsteroidal product of the germinal epithelium called "inhibin" appears to contribute to FSH regulation. Normally, infants show increases in both FSH and LH during the first months of life, which then decline to low levels until puberty. It is probable that gonadal secretions are responsible for the decline, since gonadotropin concentrations are higher in castrate patients throughout childhood.[14] In one series of 96 children with undescended testes, 79.2% had normal basal LH concentrations, whereas 20.8% had increased levels that did not correlate with testosterone concentrations.[11] Other authors reported a lower urinary LH excretion in bilateral cases from ages six to 7.9 years[12] or deficiencies in the LH responses to LH-RH with normal basal levels. These studies suggest that testosterone may not be the only factor responsible for the negative feedback control of LH. Finally, some investigators found normal levels of FSH in the basal state and after LH-RH administration in cryptorchidism,[15] whereas others demonstrated increased FSH responses to LH-RH but normal LH responses.[16] In this latter study, the abnormality in FSH correlated with the number of spermatogonia observed on testicular biopsy, suggesting a relationship between a product of the seminiferous tubules and FSH even in the prepubertal child.

Most of these studies conclude that cryptorchidism is a herterogeneous condition and that, in some cases, these abnormalities were primary and responsible for the failure of testicular descent, whereas in others an intrinsic or developing abnormality of the malpositioned gonad alters factors other than testosterone that produce changes of hypothalamic regulation even before puberty.

At puberty the sensitivity of the hypothalamic receptor sites to the feedback suppressive effects of gonadal sex steroids declines. Larger amounts of gonadotropin are secreted, first in a nocturnal pattern, and then throughout the 24-hour period until gonadal function establishes a new feedback equilibrium.[17] In the male, testicular androgenic secretion is augmented and responsible for secondary sexual maturation. Testicular volume increases at the first physical sign of puberty followed by staged morphological and genital changes.[18] The process takes four or five years and is influenced by genetic, racial, socioeconomic, and environmental factors. Both cross-sectional and longitudinal studies are available that define the relationships between the secondary sexual changes and increased testicular hormonal secretion. Studies also are available that correlate increasing testicular volume through puberty with chronological age, bone age, Tanner pubic hair staging, and peak height velocity.[19]

Since cryptorchidism is a heterogeneous condition ranging from anorchism or bilateral severe morphological abnormalities of the gonads to unilateral cases where minimal abnormalities can be discerned, pubertal and postpuberal androgenic function must be defined for specific conditions. Similarly, some studies are designed to assess testicular function in adults who were surgically treated for cryptorchidism in childhood, whereas others investigate androgenic function in untreated patients.

In unilateral cryptorchidism, both before and after surgery, compensatory testicular hypertrophy of the original scrotal gonad is often detected.[20] Clinically puberty progresses normally, and basal testosterone concentrations are essentially normal. However, when evaluated relative to the stages of puberty, even higher than normal concentrations of testosterone can be detected in the earlier stages.[21] The mechanism appears to be secondary to augmented secretion of FSH, which may be increased as a result of reduced inhibitory activity from the normal gonad.[22] The FSH may not only increase Sertoli cells[22] but also sensitize the Leydig cells to endogenous LH, producing additional testosterone.[23] When these patients are evaluated as adults, basal testosterone concentrations continue to be normal, as does virilization. However, the abnormally high FSH concentrations persist, and abnormalities in semen production and sperm count are frequently detected.[24]

In bilateral cryptorchidism the results of hormonal measurements suggest a spectrum of testicular damage, although in postsurgical patients it is impossible to determine whether the defects stem from the disorder or the treatment. However, although absolute testosterone deficiency is rarely seen,[25] azospermia and oligospermia are frequent findings.[26] These and other studies confirm that if cryptorchidism is not associated with pituitary disease, chromosomal abnormalities, or complex genetic syndromes, function is maintained in all but the most severe cases of testicular aplasia or anorchism.

CONGENITAL ANORCHISM: VANISHING TESTIS SYNDROME

Failure to locate testes in an otherwise normal boy has been reported to occur in one of 35,000 male infants.[27] These infants have normally masculinized external genitalia at birth; if exploratory laparotomy is performed, paired masculine sex accessory structures are found and müllerian structures are absent. Based on the experiments of Jost as well as on subsequent series on müllerian inhibiting substance of Sertoli cell origin, fetal testicular activity must have been present at least up to 100 days. Why the gonads subsequently vanish is obscure in most cases. Intrauterine torsion, infarction, infection, or impairment of vascular supply during testicular descent have all been proposed as mechanisms.

Inasmuch as this condition mimics bilateral cryptorchidism, several endocrinologic manipulations have been used in an attempt to distinguish it and spare the patient an extensive abdominal exploration. Failure of a plasma testosterone rise following exogenous administration of HCG, elevated levels of FSH at puberty,[27] and an augmented LH response to LH-RH at the normal age for puberty have all been investigated. Presumably studies in neonates also would fail to show a plasma testosterone surge, and plasma gonadotropin levels might be elevated as well. The various tests designed to distinguish this condition from bilateral cryptorchidism are discussed in Chapter 12. Functionally, however, anorchism does not give rise to a clinically androgen-deficient state until puberty. At that time, failure of secondary sexual characteristics to develop would become evident. Similarly, the adolescent growth spurt and resulting epiphyseal fusion would not occur, so that growth would progress at a steady rather than an accelerated rate and ultimately produce eunuchoid proportions. Thus the body habitus of the hypogonadal male could evolve as follows: facial hair would be minimal and the hairline would not recede; laryngeal development and notching would not occur, nor would the consequent deepening of the voice; axillary and pubic hair, which grows as a consequence of both gonadal and adrenal androgens, would be diminished without attaining a male escutcheon; the phallus would remain unstimulated, as would the prostate; muscle strength would be lacking; and increased truncal and hip adiposity would be expected.[28]

Obviously, untreated hypogonadism is rare, and this condition should not be allowed to develop as a consequence of anorchism or severe gonadal dysfunction. If the diagnosis has been established prior to the normal time for puberty (11 to 12 years), therapy is not initiated until this time. If diagnosed later, therapy is begun after the diagnostic studies have been completed.

There are several protocols for androgen replacement therapy. When started early (age 11 to 12 years), a gradually increasing dosage schedule should be followed in an attempt to mimic the normal stages of puberty. This may be done first with orally administered androgen, followed by intramuscular injection of long-acting preparations when higher dosages are reached. Currently, however, the types of testosterone preparations that should be employed are under scrutiny. Although rare, longer-term use of anabolic steroids has been associated with various hepatic disorders including cholestasis, cystic transfor-

TABLE 8-1.—TREATMENT OF ANDROGEN DEFICIENCY

AGE (YR)	PREPARATION	ROUTE	DOSAGE
11-13	Testosterone propionate	Buccal	5-10 mg/da
	Methyl testosterone	Buccal	5-10 mg/da
	Methyl testosterone	Oral	10-25 mg/da
13-15	Testosterone propionate	Buccal	10-20 mg/da
	Methyl testosterone	Buccal	10-20 mg/da
	Testosterone enanthate in oil	IM°	50-100 mg every 2-3 wk
15 to adult	Testosterone enanthate in oil	IM°	100-200 mg every 2-3 wk

°IM = intramuscularly.

mation (peliosis hepatis), and primary liver tumors. The most frequent association has been with orally administered 17-alkylated compounds, e.g., methyltestosterone and oxymetholone, although there is a suggestion that other steroids could cause similar toxicity.[29, 30] It is unclear whether the problem is related to dosage, to underlying hepatic disease, or to the route of administration (oral; directly through the portal circulation to the liver as opposed to the buccal route; into the systemic venous circulation; or intramuscular, also introduced into the systemic circulation). These questions are still unanswered, but the need for androgen replacement is unquestionable. We are currently using the preparations and doses outlined in Table 8-1. In the future, it is anticipated that non-17α derivatives, either testosterone ester or L-methyl DHT, will be available for long-term oral use.

REFERENCES
1. Jost A.: A new look at the mechanisms controlling sex differentiation in mammals. *Johns Hopkins Med. J.* 130:38, 1972.
2. Donahoe P.K., Ito Y., Marfaha S.R., et al.: The range of activity of müllerian inhibiting substance. *Pediatr. Res.* 9:4, 1975.
3. Blanchard M.G., Josso N.: Source of the anti-müllerian hormone synthesized by the fetal testis: Müllerian-inhibiting activity of fetal bovine Sertoli cells in tissue culture. *Pediatr. Res.* 8:968, 1974.
4. Federman D.D.: *Abnormal Sexual Development: A Genetic and Endocrine Approach to Differential Diagnosis.* Philadelphia, W.B. Saunders Co., 1967.
5. Imperato-McGinley J., Peterson R.E.: Male pseudohermaphroditism: The complexities of male phenotypic development. *Am. J. Med.* 61:251, 1976.
6. Reyes F.I., Winter J.S.D., Faiman C.: Gonadotropin-gonadal interrelationships in the fetus, in *Diabetes and Other Endocrine Disorders During Pregnancy and Newborn.* New York, Alan R. Liss, Inc., 1976.
7. Forest M.G., Sizonenko P.C., Cathiard A.M., et al.: Hypophysio-gonadal

function in humans during the first year of life: 1. Evidence for testicular activity in early infancy. *J. Clin. Invest.* 53:819, 1974.

8. Job J.C., Gendrel D., Safar A., et al.: Pituitary LH and FSH and testosterone secretion in infants with undescended testes. *Acta Endocrinol.* 85: 644, 1977.

9. Ducharme J.R., Forest M.G., DePeretti F., et al.: Plasma adrenal and gonadal sex steroids in human pubertal development. *J. Clin. Endocrinol. Metab.* 42:468, 1976.

10. Gupta D., Attanasio A., Raaf S.: Plasma estrogens and androgen concentrations in children during adolescence. *J. Clin. Endocrinol. Metab.* 40: 636, 1975.

11. Koch H., Rahlf G.: Endocrinologic and morphologic investigations on 208 prepubertal, pubertal and postpubertal patients with cryptorchidism. *Acta Endocrinol.* 193[suppl.]:85, 1975.

12. Waaler P.E.: Endocrinological studies in undescended testes. *Acta Paediatr. Scand.* 65:559, 1976.

13. Aynsley-Green A., Zachmann M., Illig R., et al.: Congenital bilateral anorchia in childhood: A clinical, endocrine and therapeutic evaluation of twenty-one cases. *Clin. Endocrinol.* 5:381, 1976.

14. Winter J.S.D., Faiman C.: Serum gonàdotropin levels in agonadal children and adults. *J. Clin. Endocrinol. Metab.* 35:561, 1972.

15. Cacciari E., Cicognani A., Pirazzoli P., et al.: Hypophyso-gonadal function in the cryptorchid child: Differences between unilateral and bilateral cryptorchids. *Acta Endocrinol.* 83:182, 1976.

16. Sizonenko P.C., Schindler A.M., Roland W., et al.: FSH: III. Evidence for a possible prepubertal regulation of its secretion by the seminiferous tubules in cryptorchid boys. *J. Clin. Endocrinol. Metab.* 46:301, 1977.

17. Root A.W.: The endocrinology of puberty. *J. Pediatr.* 83:1, 1973.

18. Tanner J.M.: *Growth at Adolescence,* ed. 2. Oxford, Blackwell Scientific Publications; Springfield, Ill., Charles C Thomas, 1965.

19. Zachmann M., Prader A., Kind H.P., et al.: Testicular volume during adolescence: Cross-sectional and longitudinal studies. *Helv. Paediatr. Acta* 29:61, 1974.

20. Laron Z., Zilka E.: Compensatory hypertrophy of testicle in unilateral cryptorchidism. *J. Clin. Endocrinol. Metab.* 29:1409, 1969.

21. Sizonenko P.C., Cuendet A., Paunier L.: FSH I. Evidence for its mediating role on testosterone secretion in cryptorchidism. *J. Clin. Endocrinol. Metab.* 37:68, 1973.

22. Laron Z., Dickerman Z., Prager-Lewin R., et al.: Plasma LH and FSH response to LRH in boys with compensatory testicular hypertrophy. *J. Clin. Endocrinol. Metab.* 40:977, 1975.

23. Cunningham G.R., Tindall D.J., Huckins C., et al.: Mechanisms for the testicular hypertrophy which follows hemi-castration. *Endocrinology* 102:16, 1978.

24. Lipshultz L.I., Caminos-Torres R., Greenspan C.G., et al.: Testicular function after orchiopexy for unilaterally undescended testis. *N. Engl. J. Med.* 295:15, 1976.

25. Bramble F.J., Ecches S., Houghton A.L., et al.: Reproductive and endocrine function after surgical treatment of bilateral cryptorchidism. *Lancet* 2:311, 1974.

26. Werder E.A., Illig R., Torresani T., et al.: Gonadal function in young adults after surgical treatment of cryptorchidism. *Br. Med. J.* 2:1357, 1976.
27. Levitt S.B., Kogan S.J., Schneider K.M., et al.: Endocrine tests in phenotypic children with bilateral impalpable testes can reliably predict "congenital" anorchism. *Urology* 11:11, 1978.
28. London D.R.: Medical aspects of hypogonadism. *Clin. Endocrinol. Metabol.* 4(3):597, 1975.
29. Westaby D., Paradinas F.J., Ogle S.J., et al.: Liver damage from long-term methyltestosterone. *Lancet* 2:261, 1977.
30. Falk H., Popper H., Thomas L.B., et al.: Hepatic angiosarcoma associated with androgenic-anabolic steroids. *Lancet* 2:1120, 1979.

9 / LH-RH Analogues and the Undescended Testis

BARRY B. BERCU, M.D.
PATRICIA K. DONAHOE, M.D.

ALTHOUGH THE PROCESS of testicular descent is still inadequately understood, the use of LH-RH in treating the undescended testis is based on an assumption that normal testicular descent requires an intact hypothalamic-pituitary-gonadal axis.[1] It is also unclear which hormones are required for descent, what end-organs or receptor-containing organs respond to produce descent, and whether these receptors vary with ontogeny. Recently Radhakrishnan et al.[2] described the morphological changes of the rat gubernaculum during embryonic development and after birth when the structure disappears. Although the gubernaculum is a likely candidate as a responsive receptor end-organ, there is no direct evidence of hormonal control on this muscular tissue. In 1938 Hamilton[3] showed that systemic testosterone caused testicular descent in the macaque monkey. Rajfer and Walsh[4, 5] recently suggested that DHT was necessary for normal descent and that gonadotropins were required to induce the 5α-reductase enzyme in the rat. Donahoe et al.[6] suggested that since most cryptorchidism is unilateral, locally active factors may be important.

As mentioned in Chapter 3, 60 XX Saanen goats have reversed male phenotypes associated with an autosomal defect, absence of horns (polled)[7]; these intersex goats tend to have asymmetric gonads with a descended testis on one side and an undescended gonad on the other. In one specimen, for example, both gonads produced testosterone but the undescended gonad had retained müllerian duct structures on the ipsilateral side, indicating absence of müllerian inhibiting substance activity, whereas the descended testis had no müllerian duct structures, indicating the presence of müllerian inhibiting substance activity. We raise the consideration that müllerian inhibiting substance may be important to normal descent of the testis.

Increased frequency of cryptorchidism in hypogonadotropic hypogonadism and a report of impaired LH-RH response in cryptorchid prepubertal boys[8] and infants[9] point to the insufficiency in the hypothalamic-pituitary-gonadal system. Functional and ultrastructural findings in estrogen-induced cryptorchidism in mice[10, 11]and in rats[5] and their prevention with HCG suggest involvement of gonadotropins in the process of descent. On the basis of these observations, Hadžiselimović et al.[12] treat cryptorchidism with HCG. Although numerous studies suggest the efficacy of HCG treatment for cryptorchidism,[1] the mechanism of action is unknown. Often the effects of treatment are temporary; several investigators believe that descent after HCG treatment, on the contrary, strongly suggests that the testis was retractile rather than cryptorchid. Failure of descent may be related to dysgenesis. Some authors hold that dysgenesis may occur in both testes, but maldescent in only one.[8, 9, 13-15]

As mentioned earlier, whether the testis fails to descend because it is dysgenic or whether it becomes abnormal as a result of its inappropriate location remains unanswered; both factors probably are important. For example, there is abundant experimental evidence in rodents and man that increasing the testicular temperature only a few degrees (42–43 C) as briefly as 30 minutes causes damage to primary spermatocytes.[16] Similar experiments in men produce oligospermia within five weeks that lasts about 50 days.[17]

Scorer and Farrington[18] believe that completion of descent cannot be evaluated until after the third postnatal month and that spontaneous descent is unlikely to occur after one year of age. The best estimates of the incidence of cryptorchidism are that 1% occurs at one year and 0.8% in adult men; however, some authors have reported a considerably higher frequency. These overestimates probably result from the failure to differentiate between retractile and undescended testes.[19] In newborn infants with undescended testes, 75% of testes descend in the first year of life and 10% in the second. However, histologic changes become apparent in the true undescended testis by age two years.[10, 11] Influenced by these factors, we suggest orchiopexy for children with cryptorchidism after one year but before age two, if the testis is truly undescended rather than retractile. A course of HCG can be used to differentiate between these two conditions. We do not yet employ LH-RH analogue treatment but are monitoring developments and will adapt our approach as the results of these studies dictate. A physician dealing with cryptorchidism should be aware of the evolving literature on the treatment of cryptorchidism with LH-RH.[20] Unlike HCG, LH-RH appears to be effective in bringing about descent

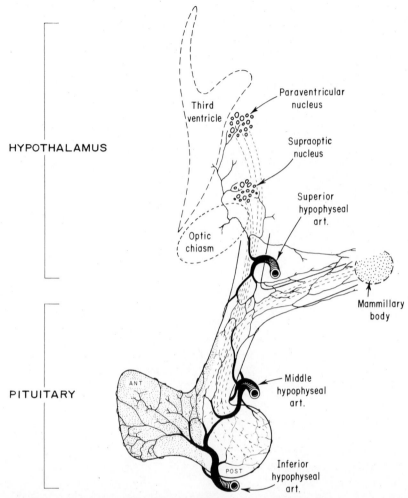

Fig 9–1.—Diagrammatic representation of hypothalamic-pituitary nervous interconnections. Bergland and Page[45] recently demonstrated complex vascular arterial and capillary interconnections between anterior and posterior pituitary and hypothalamus, thus allowing pituitary hormones to directly affect hypothalamus and brain.

of the inguinal and abdominal testis rather than the retractile inguinal testis alone.

Green and Harris[21] in 1947 first suggested that the hypothalamus might control pituitary hormones. Sawyer et al.[22] in 1949 more specifically proposed that the CNS controlled gonadotropin release, since external influences such as season, light, nutrition, and emotional stress had long been known to influence reproduction and sexual function. Figure 9–1 diagrammatically portrays the vascular and nervous interrelations of the hypothalamus and pituitary. Saffran and Schally[23] later demonstrated (1955) the existence of a hypothalamic releasing factor when crude extracts of the hypothalamus added to anterior pituitary slices in vitro caused release of ACTH. Although corticotropin-releasing factor itself has never been isolated, full-scale purification procedures of porcine pituitaries by Schally[24] and of bovine pituitaries by Guillemin,[25] as recently reviewed in their respective Nobel laureate addresses, led to the isolation and purification of thyrotropin-releasing hormone (TRH) and subsequently LH-RH, a decapeptide that is responsible for the release of both LH and FSH from the pituitary. Using hundreds of thousands of hypothalami, LH-RH was purified and sequenced (Glu-His-Trp-Ser-Tyr-Gly-Leu-Arg-Pro-Gly). Guillemin and Schally and their co-workers then synthesized LH-RH, demonstrating LH and FSH release both in vivo and in vitro. The bioactivity of the synthetic product was identical to that of the previously purified natural product.

During the past several years, more than 1,000 analogues (agonists and antagonists) have been synthesized using rapid solid-phase techniques. Figure 9–2 reviews the modifications that have been made in the parent molecule to produce the potent analogues used to treat patients with cryptorchidism. Substitution at position 6 or 10 yields more potent and prolonged agonist activity.[26] Vale et al.[26] suggest that LH-RH has certain amino acid positions essential for receptor binding and biologic activity, as well as others necessary to maintain the tertiary structure of the molecule, probably facilitating a stable conformation and easy recognition. Highly active analogues have been obtained by substitution of Gly^6 with a D-amino acid where the molecule makes a U turn, and replacement of the N-terminal glycinamide (Gly^{10}) by alkylamines, producing LH-RH nonapeptides. These modifications contribute to stability against inactivating enzymes.[27]

When given frequently, pharmacologic doses of LH-RH can have paradoxical effects and impair reproductive function; the mechanisms for these phenomena are unknown. Long-term administration of LH-RH or agonists has been shown in the female to cause cessation of cycling and atrophy of the ovaries and uterus.[28] Other studies have shown effects on male rat gonads, with a reduction of both testicular receptors and circulating testosterone levels.[29] Recent in vitro data suggest that these effects may be extrapituitary, occurring because of direct effects of LH-RH on the peripheral tissue rather than on the

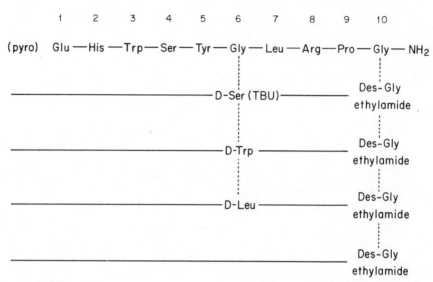

Fig 9-2.—LH-RH parent molecule. Substitution of glycine in position 6 with a D amino acid such as serine, tryptophan, or leucine, and/or replacement of N-terminal glycine by ethylamide, has produced potent nonapeptide analogues used to treat cryptorchidism. *TBU* = tertiary butyl ether.

pituitary gland. Indeed, early in gestation, LH-RH in large doses can block implantation[30-35] and terminate pregnancy in rats; late in gestation, it can delay parturition.[36] LH-RH appears to have a direct effect on steroidogenesis in both the testis and ovary.[29, 36, 37] As a result of these extrapituitary actions, caution must be exercised in devising clinical protocols for these drugs.

To avoid the paradoxical effect of LH-RH on gonadotropin secretion, investigators have varied the time schedule of dose administration. Besser[38] and Crowley[39] have successfully treated hypogonadotropic hypogonadal men with LH-RH analogues. However, the dosage and frequency of administering the LH-RH analogues have proved to be critical variables in establishing or extinguishing pituitary responsiveness in these patients. Crowley first met with success by changing the daily dosage to treatment on every other day and, based on Knobil's observations, is now using small-bolus hourly doses. Knobil et al.[41] carefully evaluated LH-RH secretion in female monkeys and observed that LH-RH secretion, as represented by LH peaks, occurs once every hour. This group is now pursuing studies on LH-RH replacement using this dosage schedule. Short and Lincoln[42] have treated animals with hourly pulses of LH-RH to produce changes in seasonal breeding behavior. From the observations of these investigators, it appears reasonable to conclude that physiologic replacement should be intermittent.

Happ et al.[43] recently treated 25 boys, ranging from one to 10 years of age, who had unilateral or bilateral cryptorchidism, by administering 200 μg of LH-RH pernasally six times a day until descent was completed, or for a maximum of 10 weeks. Complete descent occurred in 16 patients, usually after two to five weeks of treatment; no adverse side effects were observed. Of 36 undescended testes (20 right, 16 left in 25 patients), treatment effected complete descent in 23 (16 right, nine left), partial descent in nine, and no change in four. There was a suggestion of reduced basal LH secretion and responsiveness, whereas no differences were seen in FSH secretion.

Twenty-two prepubertal children with unilaterally undescended testis were treated with 200 μg of LH-RH six times a day (1,200 μg/24 hours) or with 500 μg twice a day (1,000 μg/24 hours) by nasal insufflation.[44] Full descent resulted in seven cases and partial but definite descent in six, i.e., 13 of 22 responses. Neither basal nor LH-RH stimulated LH or FSH levels varied between control and therapeutic groups.

The use of LH-RH analogues as demonstrated by these studies may provide an important pharmacologic approach to patients with cryptorchidism. Careful consideration must be given to these compounds, but caution must be exercised until more is known about their side effects and until appropriate dosage and time schedules of administration are developed.

REFERENCES

1. Hadžiselimović F.: Cryptorchidism and ultrastructure of normal and cryptorchid testis development. *Adv. Anat. Embryol. Cell Biol.* 53(3):72, 1977.
2. Radhakrishnan J., Morikawa Y., Donahoe P.K., et al.: Observations on the gubernaculum during descent of the testis. *Invest. Urol.* 16:365, 1979.
3. Hamilton J.B.: The effect of male hormone upon the descent of the testes. *Anat. Rec.* 70:533, 1938.
4. Rajfer J., Walsh P.C.: Hormonal regulation of testicular descent: Experimental and clinical observations. *J. Urol.* 118:985, 1977.
5. Rajfer J., Walsh P.C.: Testicular descent. *Birth Defects* 13:107, 1977.
6. Donahoe P.K., Ito Y., Morikawa Y., et al.: Müllerian inhibiting substance in human testes after birth. *J. Pediatr. Surg.* 12:323, 1977.
7. Short R.V., Hamerton J.L., Grieves S.A., et al.: An intersex goat with bilaterally asymmetrical reproductive tract. *J. Reprod. Fertil.* 16:283, 1968.
8. Job J.C., Garnier P.E., Chaussain J.L., et al.: Effect of synthetic luteiniz-

ing hormone-releasing hormone on the release of gonadotropins in hypophysogonadal disorders of children and adolescents. IV. Undescended testes. *J. Pediatr.* 84:371, 1974.

9. Job J.C., Gendrel D., Safar A., et al.: Pituitary LH and FSH and testosterone secretion in infants with undescended testes. *Acta Endocrinol. (Copenh.)* 85:644, 1977.

10. Hadžiselimović F., Herzog B.: The meaning of the Leydig cell in relation to the etiology of cryptorchidism: An experimental electronmicroscopic study. *J. Pediatr. Surg.* 11:1, 1976.

11. Hadžiselimović F., Girard J.: Cryptorchidism: Ultrastructure of normal and cryptorchid testis development. *Adv. Anat. Embryol. Cell. Biol.* 53: 53, 1977.

12. Hadžiselimović F., Girard, J., Herzog B.: Treatment of cryptorchidism by synthetic luteinizing hormone-releasing hormone. *Lancet* 2:1125, 1977.

13. Sohval A.R.: Histopathology of cryptorchidism: A study based upon the comparative histology of retained and scrotal testes from birth to maturity. *Am. J. Med.* 16:346, 1954.

14. Charney C.W.: The spermatogenic potential of the undescended testis before and after treatment. *J. Urol.* 83:697, 1960.

15. Johnston J.H.: The undescended testis. *Arch. Dis. Child.* 40:113, 1965.

16. Steinberger E., Dixon W.J.: Some observations on the effect of heat on the testicular germinal epithelium. *Fertil. Steril.* 10:578, 1959.

17. MacLeod J., Hotchkiss R.S.: The effect of hyperpyrexia upon spermatozoa counts in men. *Endocrinology* 28:780, 1941.

18. Scorer C.G., Farrington G.H.: The testis at birth and during infancy, in *Congenital Deformities of the Testis and Epididymis.* New York, Appleton-Century-Crofts, 1971, p. 15.

19. Sherins R.J., Howards S.S.: Male infertility, in *Campbell's Textbook of Urology.* Philadelphia, W.B. Saunders Co., 1978, p. 715.

20. Sandon J.: *Basic Applications and Clinical Uses of Hypothalamic Hormones.* Amsterdam, Excerpta Medica, 1976, p. 113.

21. Green J.D., Harris G.W.: The neurovascular link between the neurohypophysis and adenohypophysis. *J. Endocrinol.* 5:136, 1947.

22. Sawyer C.H., Everett J.W., Markee J.E.: A neural factor in the mechanism by which estrogen induces the release of luteinizing hormone in the rat. *Endocrinology* 44:218, 1949.

23. Saffran M., Schally A.V.: The release of corticotropin by anterior pituitary tissue in vitro. *Can. J. Biochem.* 33:408, 1955.

24. Schally A.V.: Aspects of hypothalamic regulation of the pituitary gland. *Science* 202:18, 1978.

25. Guillemin R.: Peptides in the brain: The new endocrinology of the neuron. *Science* 202:390, 1978.

26. Vale W., Rivier C., Brown M., et al.: Pharmacology of thyrotropin releasing factor (TRF), luteinizing hormone releasing factor (LRF), and somatostatin, in Porter J.C. (ed.): *Hypothalamic Peptide Hormones and Pituitary Regulation.* New York, Plenum Press, 1977.

27. Marks N., Stern F.: Enzymatic mechanisms for the inactivation of luteinizing hormone-releasing hormone (LH-RH). *Biochem. Biophys. Res. Commun.* 61:1458, 1974.

28. Corbin A., Beattie C.W., Tracy J., et al.: The anti-reproductive pharmacology of LH-RH and agonistic analogues. *Int. J. Fertil.* 23:81, 1978.
29. Hseuh A.J.W.: Extrapituitary action of gonadotropin-releasing hormone (GnRH): Direct inhibition of ovarian and testicular responses. 61st Annual Meeting of the Endocrine Society, Anaheim, Calif., 1979, Abst. 198.
30. Lin Y.C.L., Yoshinaga K.: Inhibitory effect on ovum implantation in the rat. 58th Annual Meeting of the Endocrine Society 1976, p. 143.
31. Beattie C.W., Corbin A., Cole G., et al.: Mechanism of the postcoital contraceptive effect of LH-RH in the rat. Serum hormone levels during chronic LH-RH administration. *Biol. Reprod.* 16:322, 1977.
32. Rippel R.H., Johnson E.S.: Regression of corpora lutea in the rabbit after injection of a gonadotropin releasing peptide. *Proc. Soc. Exp. Biol. Med.* 152:29, 1976.
33. Humphrey R.R., Windsor B.L., Reel J.R., et al.: The effects of luteinizing hormone-releasing hormone (LH-RH) in pregnant rats. I. Postnidatory effects. *Biol. Reprod.* 16:614, 1977.
34. Humphrey R.R., Windsor B.L., Jones D.C., et al.: The progesterone-sensitive period of rat pregnancy: Some effects of LH-RH and ovariectomy. *Proc. Soc. Biol. Med.* 156:345, 1977.
35. MacDonald G.J., Beattie C.W.: Pregnancy failure in hypophysectomized rats following LH-RH administration. *Life Sci.* 24:1103, 1979.
36. Bercu B.B., Hayashi A., Poth M., et al.: LH-RH induced delay of parturition. IV International Congress of Endocrinology, Melbourne, Australia, Feb. 1980.
37. Hseuh A.J.W., Erickson G.F.: Extrapituitary action of gonadotropin-releasing hormone: Direct inhibition of ovarian steroidogenesis. *Science* 204:854, 1979.
38. Besser G.M., McNeilly A.S., Anderson D.C., et al.: Hormonal responses to synthetic luteinizing hormone and follicle stimulating hormone-releasing hormone in man. *Br. Med. J.* 3:267, 1972.
39. Crowley W.: Chronic administration of a long acting LRF agonist (D-Trp⁶-Pro⁹-Net-LRF) in hypogonadotropic hypogonadism: The critical nature of dosage and frequency in enhancement, extinction, and restoration. 61st Annual Meeting of the Endocrine Society, Anaheim, Calif., 1979, Abst. 16.
40. Belchetz P.E., Plant T.M., Nakai Y., et al.: Hypophyseal responses to continuous and intermittent delivery of hypothalamic gonadotropin releasing hormone. *Science* 202:631, 1978.
41. Knobil E., Plant T.: Hypothalamic control of the primate menstrual cycle. *Recent Prog. Horm. Res.* 36:1980.
42. Short R.V., Lincoln G.A.: Seasonal breeding: Nature's contraceptive. *Recent Prog. Horm. Res.* 36:1980.
43. Happ J., Kollmann F., Draivehl C., et al.: Treatment of cryptorchidism with pernasal gonadotropin-releasing hormone therapy. *Fertil. Steril.* 29:546, 1978.
44. Pirazzoli P., Zappulla F., Bernard F., et al.: Luteinizing hormone-releasing hormone nasal spray as therapy for undescended testicle. *Arch. Dis. Child.* 53:235, 1978.
45. Bergland R.M., Page R.B.: Pituitary-brain vascular relations: A new paradigm. *Science* 204:18, 1979.

10 / Complications of Cryptorchidism

ERIC W. FONKALSRUD, M.D.

FAILURE OF NORMAL testicular descent has many disadvantages, perhaps the most important of which is that when the testis remains in the elevated temperature of the body wall sufficiently long, normal maturation and subsequent spermatogenic function become severely retarded (see Chapter 6). Also of great concern is the undisputed role that cryptorchidism plays in testicular tumorigenesis (see Chapter 13).

The scrotal temperature in human beings ranges between 1.5 and 3 C lower than that in the abdomen. In 1921 Crew[1] demonstrated that testicular degeneration may result from prolonged exposure to the higher surrounding temperature of the abdomen. Piana[2] in 1891 and Moore et al.[3, 4] in 1924 produced experimental cryptorchidism by surgically transferring the testis from the scrotum to the abdomen, demonstrating intratubular epithelial degeneration identical to that observed in natural cryptorchidism. Further studies showed that heating the scrotum with externally applied warming techniques caused degenerative changes in the seminiferous tubules similar to those seen in cryptorchid gonads. Moreover, it was demonstrated that placing scrotal testes into the abdomen causes degeneration of germinal epithelium and that normal germinal maturation recurred within three to six months when the testes were returned to the scrotum.[5] Similar studies by Kiesewetter et al.[6] have shown that when a mature puppy testis is placed into the abdominal wall, the testis loses weight and its tubular architecture is markedly altered. Recent studies by Robinson et al.[7] have shown that the human sperm count may be lowered substantially by exposing the scrotum for short intervals to heat from a light bulb during a two-week period, whereas cooling the scrotum with an ice bag increases the sperm count significantly and thus can be used clinically to treat infertility.

It is therefore generally accepted that the scrotum and cremaster mechanism serve as a thermoregulator for the testis and that the degeneration of seminiferous tubules apparent in cryptorchid gonads stems partly from their location in a region of higher temperature. This concept, which is further supported by evidence of tubular degeneration subsequent to prolonged febrile illness in men[8] and after scrotal insulating experiments,[9] has provided the rationale for therapeutic placement of the cryptorchid testis into the scrotum. However, this line of reasoning fails to explain why the contralateral descended testis often shows abnormal morphologic characteristics.

DECREASED SPERMATOGENIC FUNCTION

It was believed for many years, based on a limited number of testicular biopsies, that the human male gonad remained in a resting stage from birth until about the fifth year of life.[10, 11] This opinion has been modified owing to recent studies by Staedtler and Hartmann[12] showing that continuous testicular growth begins immediately after birth, as indicated by an increase in testicular size, tubular diameter, and the number of spermatogonia (see Chapter 6). It has been suggested that spermatogonia content, apart from tubular maturation, is the crucial measurement when assessing impairment of function of the undescended testes.[13, 14]

In perhaps the most comprehensive study of testicular biopsy specimens, Mengel et al.[13] examined tissue from 515 undescended and 237 unilaterally descended testes. They found that most unilaterally cryptorchid testes have normal morphologic features and spermatogonia content during the first two years of life. However, gonads that remain out of the scrotum by the beginning of the third year have a statistically significant decrease in spermatogonia content and tubular growth. Hadžiselimović et al.[15] similarly observed no ultrastructural differences in the seminiferous tubules between scrotal and undescended testes up to the age of one year, but after that time significant differences were noted. Further studies demonstrated that the rate and number of cells involved and DNA synthesis in cryptorchid testes are markedly inferior to those of the contralateral descended gonad.[16]

Possibly the most significant complication of cryptorchidism is the failure of the seminiferous tubules to mature normally and the resulting inability of the gonad to produce normal mature sperm. Much of the literature on this subject during the past three decades has dealt with the time when degenerative changes in seminiferous tubule structure occur in cryptorchid testes. Opinions are widely diversified on this matter; some authors indicate that the undescended testis is abnormal at birth or becomes so shortly thereafter,[17] whereas others maintain that the cryptorchid testis does not show degenerative changes until shortly before adolescence.[18, 19] Most recent studies,

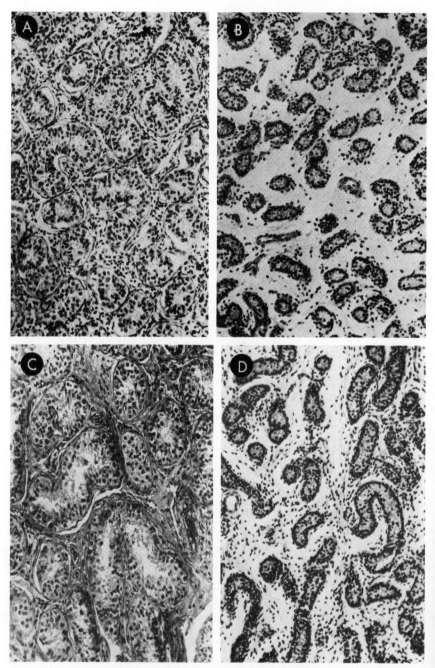

Fig 10–1. — See legend on facing page.

however, claim that although slight histologic differences between normal and cryptorchid testes may exist during the first two years of life, there is evidence of progressive severe degenerative changes in the nonscrotal testis after the age of two to five years (Fig 10–1).[11, 20, 21] The difficulty in interpreting these disparate observations occurs partly because many authors have not indicated the degree of undescent of the testis as defined by Scorer[22] and because the studies usually have represented a wide age range. An extensive review of the subject has been published by Levin and Sherman.[23]

The tubular fertility index (percentage of testicular tubules seen to contain spermatogonia, TFI) devised by Mack et al.[24] compares the germinal cell content of testes from different patients and is more reliable than comparing the mean diameter of the seminiferous tubules, as was done previously. After reviewing more than 265 testicular biopsies, Farrington[25] showed that complete spermatogenesis was evident by the 15th year in all normal as well as unilaterally descended testes. Testes of normal males have a TFI of 100% by the age of 15 years, but the level in cryptorchid testes remains at about 25%, with no increase in late adolescence. The TFI appears to correlate closely with the degree of descent of the testis[25]; gonads at the scrotal neck have a TFI of 42.4%; those in the superficial inguinal pouch, 31.5%; those in the inguinal canal, 19.1%; and intra-abdominal testes, 4.8%. In many males the unilaterally descended testis both commences and completes spermatogenesis at an earlier age than does the normal testis, indicating a degree of hyperplasia, possibly to compensate for the deficiency in the undescended testis. A small proportion (4%) of the unilaterally descended testes showed tubular dysgenesis in Farrington's study,[25] whereas the remainder appeared to have a capability for normal spermatogenesis at puberty.

A somewhat more pessimistic view concerning the function of the unilaterally descended testis was presented by Hecker and Hienz,[10] who reviewed biopsies from both testes in 125 patients with unilateral cryptorchidism. They found that although dystopic testes never ma-

---

Fig 10–1.—**A,** normal testis from six-year-old boy in active growth phase showing evidence of tubular enlargement and cellular differentiation. **B,** six-year-old testis showing no evidence of growth. Interstitial edema illustrates effect of exogenous HCG administration. **C,** testis from normal 11-year-old boy showing tubular enlargement and cellular differentiation compared to **A.** Leydig's cells are present. **D,** testis from 10-year-old cryptorchid boy showing severe maturation arrest and considerable interstitial fibrosis. (Reprinted by permission from Cohn, B.C.[21])

tured beyond stage II of maturation, the contralateral descended testes matured normally in only 40% of patients. These authors also noted that in 6% of patients, the degenerative changes were even more pronounced in the scrotal than in the contralateral undescended testis. Lipshultz et al.[26] noted, in a study of men over age 21 who had undergone orchiopexy for unilateral undescent 10 or more years previously, that almost all had decreased spermatogenesis, an indication that the contralateral descended testis was abnormal in all patients. In summarizing six published reports, Hecker and Hienz[10] observed that of 346 patients with uncorrected unilateral dystopia, the sperm counts of only 120 (35%) were sufficient to produce fertility. This does not, however, take into account the patients' wide age range and the varying degrees of sexual activity. Representing a somewhat extreme position, Hecker[27] has suggested that a cryptorchid testis may adversely affect the contralateral descended testis, and that in patients beyond the age of five years, orchiectomy rather than orchiopexy should be performed. Studies by Mengel and Zimmermann (see Chapter 17) have shown that when one canine testis is placed into the abdomen, the contralateral descended testis may later develop degenerative changes. A more detailed review of the results of treatment for undescent on spermatogenic function is presented in Chapter 21.

HERNIA

The peritoneum from the lower abdomen normally descends with the testis through the inguinal canal and into the scrotum to form the eventual tunica vaginalis. The narrow processus vaginalis that communicates between the tunica and the peritoneal cavity usually stretches, becoming compressed by the abdominal wall musculature in the inguinal canal, causing its obliteration within the first few weeks of life in most normal males. It is not surprising, therefore, that when the testis is arrested in its normal descent, the factors usually causing closure of the patent processus do not become effective. This in turn results in persistence of the processus, which in most patients is sufficiently large to be classified as a hernia, but only when the processus is large enough to permit abdominal contents to enter can it properly be termed a hernia. Although wide variations in the incidence of indirect inguinal hernia accompanying cryptorchidism have been reported, they may be explained in part by a difference in definition. At one extreme McCutcheon[28] found a 2% incidence in 204 cryptorchid males, whereas at the other extreme, Kiesewetter[29] reported a 97.7% incidence in 500 patients. Most authors indicate an incidence of accompanying hernia greater than 65%.[30-34] On the other hand, the coincident occurrence of a hydrocele with an undescended testis is extremely uncommon. Femoral and direct inguinal hernias also are rare in boys who have cryptorchid testes.

In some patients the hernia may be so symptomatic that it must be repaired during the first several months of life, even though the delicate nature of the spermatic cord structures makes this a suboptimal time for orchiopexy. Although herniorrhaphy is often delayed for a few months in patients with minimally symptomatic hernias,[35] the trend toward elective orchiopexy between the ages of two and four years is reflected in the fact that pediatric surgeons generally repair almost all clinically symptomatic hernias in cryptorchid males when diagnosed, regardless of age. This view also is supported by the observation that symptomatic hernias often cause testicular swelling that may further compromise the function of an already abnormal gonad. Although cryptorchidism per se usually is asymptomatic,[36] the presence of an associated hernia may produce inguinal pain. If a cryptorchid male undergoes repair of a symptomatic hernia, the testes should simultaneously be placed into the scrotum, inasmuch as subsequent spontaneous descent is unlikely, and later reoperation in a scarred wound may risk serious injury to the testicular blood supply.

TORSION OF THE UNDESCENDED TESTES

Torsion of the spermatic cord is an axial rotation or twisting of the cord upon itself, with a sudden (or sometimes gradual) constriction of the blood supply to the testis, epididymis, and investing structures. Although the condition is uncommon, a significant number of such patients are reported to be cryptorchid.[37-40] Among 150 cases of torsion, Wallenstein[41] found 90 with undescended testes. When torsion occurs in a cryptorchid testis, a nonviable gonad is more likely to result than if torsion occurs in a noncryptorchid testis.[42] The higher incidence of nonviability may possibly stem from increased difficulty in diagnosing torsion in a nonscrotal testis and perhaps is another reason to favor early orchiopexy. Hand,[43] however, reported only three instances of torsion among 153 cryptorchid patients who were observed up to 33 years. An abnormal gubernacular attachment of the testis to the scrotum[44] and of the cremaster muscle to the gonad[45] has been cited as a possible etiologic factor in torsion; however, the actual mechanism remains unclear. The true relationship of torsion to testicular undescent is not known, since almost all gonads that undergo torsion are located within the scrotum. Moreover, it is rarely necessary to perform a concomitant complete orchiopexy with retroperitoneal dissection to lengthen the cord enough to permit placing the detorsed gonad into the lower scrotum. A patient who has unilateral testicular torsion is far more likely to have torsion of the contralateral gonad at a later time, regardless of the level of descent, than is the normal male. Therefore, most surgeons perform an inguinal or, if feasible, a transscrotal pexy of the contralateral gonad, as well as formal orchiopexy of the torsed testis, if necessary, under the same anesthetic.

Torsion occasionally occurs in an undescended testis that has undergone malignant degeneration. Among cases of torsion reported in adult cryptorchid testes, 64% were found to be malignant.[46] Abeshouse[40] observed that five of 69 patients who had testicular torsion also had malignant tumors. Torsion in an undescended testis has been observed in a neonate seen clinically with an abdominal mass.[47] Torsion also may occur in utero, in which case the infarcted testis may calcify.[48] For these reasons, testicular torsion must be considered a serious indication that the cryptorchid testis should be surgically positioned into the scrotum and anchored there.

TRAUMA

A cryptorchid testis lying in the inguinal canal is more vulnerable to trauma than is the normally descended gonad because the relatively rigid abdominal wall does not afford the cushioning provided by the soft, elastic scrotum.[49] Furthermore, contraction of the abdominal muscles subjects the cryptorchid testis lodged in the inguinal canal to repeated alterations in pressure, which under certain circumstances may be traumatic and painful. Similarly, a testis lying in the superficial inguinal pouch or an ectopic gonad near the pubis often is exposed to direct and recurrent trauma. Some authors[50, 51] have suggested that repeated testicular trauma may be an etiologic factor in the frequent relationship between malignancy and cryptorchidism; however, little substantive evidence supports this view, particularly since the well-protected intra-abdominal testes are the most prone to develop a tumor.

PSYCHOLOGIC FACTORS

An empty scrotum may be a source of considerable anxiety and embarrassment, often causing feelings of physical inferiority and concern about virility.[52] Although not considered significant until the boy is exposed to peer scrutiny during early adolescence when showering in a locker room environment, some recent psychiatric studies reveal that boys at three years of age or younger may become aware that their genitalia appear different from those of their friends.[53] Their concern resembles that experienced by uncircumcised boys in the United States today who become keenly aware that most of their friends have a different appearance, although the reverse is true in many other countries.

Further anxiety is often expressed by patients and parents regarding the possibility of sterility. Assurance from the physician of the high likelihood of eventual fertility and virility in patients with unilateral undescent, after proper management, helps substantially to alleviate these well-founded anxieties. Awareness of the psychologic concerns caused by an empty scrotum has prompted the routine use of Silastic scrotal prostheses for patients who lack or have an atrophic testis.

REFERENCES

1. Crew F.A.E.: A suggestion as to the cause of the aspermatic condition of the imperfectly descended testis. *J. Anat.* 56:98, 1921.
2. Piana L., cited by Charney D.W., Wolgin W.: *Cryptorchidism.* New York, Hoeber Medical Division, Harper & Row, 1957.
3. Moore C.R.: Properties of gonads as controllers of somatic characteristics; heat application and testicular degeneration; function of the scrotum. *Am. J. Anat.* 34:337, 1924.
4. Moore C.R., Quick W.J.: The scrotum as a temperature regulator for the testes. *Am. J. Physiol.* 68:70, 1924.
5. Moore C.R.: The biology of mammalian testes and scrotum. *Q. Rev. Biol.* 1:4, 1926.
6. Kiesewetter W.B., Kalayoglu M., Sachs B.: The effect of abnormal position, scrotal repositioning, and human gonadotropic hormone on the developing puppy testis. *J. Pediatr. Surg.* 8:739, 1973.
7. Robinson D., Rock J., Menkin M.F.: Control of human spermatogenesis by induced changes of intrascrotal temperature. *J.A.M.A.* 204:80, 1968.
8. Wangensteen O.H.: Undescended testis; experimental and clinical study. *Arch. Surg.* 14:663, 1927.
9. MacLeod J., Hotchkiss R.S.: The effect of hyperpyrexia upon the spermatozoa counts in men. *Endocrinology* 28:780, 1941.
10. Hecker W., Hienz H.A.: Cryptorchidism and fertility. *J. Pediatr. Surg.* 2:513, 1967.
11. Robinson J.N., Engle E.T.: Some observations on the cryptorchid testis. *J. Urol.* 71:726, 1954.
12. Staedtler F., Hartmann R.: Histological and morphological studies of prepubertal testicular development in normal and in cerebrally damaged boys. *Dtsch. Med. Wochenschr.* 97:104, 1972.
13. Mengel W., Hienz H.A., Sippe W.G., et al.: Studies on cryptorchidism: A comparison of histological findings in the germinative epithelium before and after the second year of life. *J. Pediatr. Surg.* 9:445, 1974.
14. Hosli P.O.: The problems connected with therapy of cryptorchidism. *Acta Urol.* 2:107, 1972.
15. Hadžiselimović F., Herzog B., Seguchi H.: Surgical correction of cryptorchidism at two years: Electron microscopic and morphologic investigation. *J. Pediatr. Surg.* 10:19, 1975.

16. Markewitz M., Lattimer J.K., Veenema R.J.: A comparative study of germ cell kinetics in the testes of children with unilateral cryptorchidism: A preliminary report. *Fertil. Steril.* 21:806, 1970.

17. Mancini R.E., Rosenberg E., Cullen N., et al.: Cryptorchid and scrotal human testes: I. Cytological, cytochemical, and quantitative studies. *J. Clin. Endocrinol. Metab.* 25:927, 1965.

18. Anderson H.: Biopsy studies in cryptorchidism. *Acta Endocrinol.* 18:567, 1955.

19. Sohval A.R.: Histopathology of cryptorchidism. *Am. J. Med.* 16:346, 1954.

20. Nelson W.O.: Mammalian spermatogenesis. *Recent Prog. Horm. Res.* 6: 29, 1951.

21. Cohn B.D.: Histology of the cryptorchid testis. *Surgery* 62:536, 1967.

22. Scorer C.G.: The descent of the testis. *Arch. Dis. Child.* 39:605, 1964.

23. Levin A., Sherman J.O.: The undescended testis. *Surg. Gynecol Obstet.* 136:473, 1973.

24. Mack W.S., Scott L.S., Ferguson-Smith N.A., et al.: Ectopic testis and true undescended testis: A histological comparison. *J. Pathol.* 82:439, 1961.

25. Farrington G.H.: Histologic observations in cryptorchidism: The congenital germinal-cell deficiency of the undescended testis. *J. Pediatr. Surg.* 4: 606, 1969.

26. Lipshultz L.E., Caminos-Torres R., Greenspan C.S., et al.: Testicular function after orchiopexy for unilaterally undescended testis. *N. Engl. J. Med.* 295:15, 1976.

27. Hecker W.C.: Neue Gesichspunkte zum Kryptorchismus-Problem. *Munch. Med. Wochenschr.* 113:1125, 1971.

28. McCutcheon A.B.: Further observations on the delayed testes. *Med. J. Aust.* 1:654, 1938.

29. Kiesewetter W.B.: Undescended testes. *W. Va. Med. J.* 52:235, 1956.

30. Gross R.E., Jewett T.C. Jr.: Surgical experiences from 1,222 operations for undescended testes. *J.A.M.A.* 160:634, 1956.

31. Snyder W.H. Jr., Chaffin L.: Surgical management of undescended testes. *J.A.M.A.* 157:129, 1955.

32. Koop C.E.: Observations on undescended testes: Significance of empty scrotum, indication for orchiopexy. *Arch. Surg.* 75:801, 1957.

33. Clatworthy H.W. Jr., Gilbert M., Clement A.: The inguinal hernia, hydrocele, and undescended testicle problem in infants and children. *Postgrad. Med. J.* 22:122, 1957.

34. Coley W.B.: Treatment of undescended or maldescended testes associated with inguinal hernia. *Ann. Surg.* 48:321, 1908.

35. Gross R.E.: *The Surgery of Infancy and Childhood: Its Principles and Techniques.* Philadelphia, W.B. Saunders Co., 1953.

36. Charney C.W., Wolgin W.: *Cryptorchidism.* New York, Hoeber Medical Division, Harper & Row, 1957.

37. Snyder W.H. Jr., Greaney E.M. Jr.: Cryptorchidism, in Mustard W., Ravitch M.M., Snyder W.H. Jr., et al. (eds.): *Pediatric Surgery,* ed. 2. Chicago, Year Book Medical Publishers, Inc., 1969.

38. Allen W.R., Brown R.B.: Torsion of the testis. *Br. Med. J.* 1:1396, 1966.

39. Taylor J.N., Gauer D.J.: Torsion of the testicle. *J. Urol.* 94:680, 1965.

40. Abeshouse B.S.: Torsion of the spermatic cord: Report of three cases and review of the literature. *Urol. Cutan. Rev.* 40:699, 1936.

41. Wallenstein S.: Torsion of an intra-abdominal testis. *J. Urol.* 21:279, 1929.
42. Leape L.: Torsion of the testis: Invitation to error. *J.A.M.A.* 200:669, 1967.
43. Hand J.R.: Treatment of undescended testis and its complications. *J.A.M.A.* 164:1185, 1957.
44. Lawless E.C., Lindner H.H.: Torsion of the spermatic cord. *Surgery* 54: 471, 1963.
45. Muschat M.: Pathologic anatomy of testicular torsion: Explanation of its mechanism. *Surg. Gynecol. Obstet.* 54:758, 1932.
46. Riegler H.C.: Torsion of intra-abdominal testis. *Surg. Clin. North Am.* 52: 371, 1972.
47. Campbell J.R., Schneider C.P.: Intrauterine torsion of an intra-abdominal testis. *Pediatrics* 57:262, 1976.
48. Cho S.K. Hamoudi A.B., Clatworthy H.W. Jr.: Infarction of an abdominal undescended testis presenting as a calcified abdominal mass in a new-born. *Radiology* 110:173, 1974.
49. Alojzy M.: Significance of biopsy research in cryptorchidism in children. *Arch. Dis. Child.* 38:170, 1963.
50. Coley W.B.: Operative treatment of undescended or maldescended testes with special reference to end-results. *Surg. Gynecol. Obstet.* 28:452, 1919.
51. Collins A.N.: Trauma and malignant testes. *Lancet* 56:139, 1936.
52. Gross R.E., Replogle R.L.: Treatment of the undescended testes. *Postgrad. Med. J.* 34:266, 1963.
53. Lattimer J.K., Smith A.M., Dougherty L.J.: The optimum time to operate for cryptorchidism. *Pediatrics* 53:96, 1974.

11 / Associated Anomalies in Undescended Testis

W. HARDY HENDREN, M.D.
HOWARD B. GINSBURG, M.D.

IN MOST CASES of undescended testis, particularly when the condition is unilateral, no other anomaly is present. However, the clinician should watch for other malformations associated with cryptorchidism. Moreover, a child may be referred for orchiopexy, especially in a bilateral case, when there is a serious underlying problem such as intersexuality.

SCREENING ROENTGENOGRAMS OF THE URINARY TRACT

It is well known that a higher than normal incidence of major urinary tract malformations occurs in boys with cryptorchidism. Nevertheless, clinicians disagree as to the wisdom of obtaining routine screening films to identify the few patients who have a significant other malformation. Obviously, although it is desirable to discover other correctable anomalies, we must avoid expensive diagnostic studies involving large numbers of patients when the yield is low.

Felton[1] screened 61 boys with cryptorchidism and discovered 13% with significant other urologic malformations. Grossman et al.[2] found that 12% of 100 boys had an associated urologic anomaly. Among 140 cryptorchid boys without urologic symptoms, Noe and Patterson[3] observed major abnormalities in three and minor deformities in eight, but because none required surgical intervention, they concluded that screening was not fruitful. Other series[4,5] concluded that routine intravenous pyelogram (IVP) screening is not indicated in boys with unilateral undescended testis. Although an IVP is likely to disclose an abnormality in about 10% of cases, there is disagreement concerning the significance of this fact; some consider the presence of horseshoe kidney or renal hypoplasia an important finding; others do not.

In our practice an IVP is obtained in boys with bilateral cryptorchidism, where the yield of pathologic features tends to be higher.
Moreover, during operation while the patient is under anesthesia, we
palpate the flanks to see if there are two kidneys—a procedure that
helps to detect the absence of a kidney and the presence of hydrone-
phrosis or a horseshoe kidney. During orchiopexy, when the cord
structures are being mobilized retroperitoneally, we always visualize
the ureter. In this way we have discovered absence of a kidney in one
patient and an obstructive megaureter in another, which was later
confirmed by IVP and then repaired.

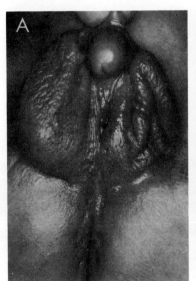 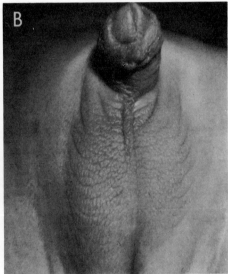

Fig 11–1.—Adrenogenital syndrome in two female infants with masculinized genitalia from adrenal cortical hyperplasia with salt-losing endocri-
nopathy. Spectrum in degree of virilization of these girls includes lower
urinary tract anatomy as well. **A,** moderate virilization, initially thought to be
hypospadias and undescended testes. In most cases, flap vaginoplasty suf-
fices because there is low confluence of vagina with urogenital sinus. Cli-
toral recession also should be performed. **B,** severe masculinization, phallus resembling normal penis in infant originally thought to be male and
named accordingly. Urethra resembled that of normal male; vagina entered
high, between external sphincter and bladder neck, at site of normal-appearing verumontanum. Reconstruction in such a severe case cannot be
accomplished by flap vaginoplasty. It requires pull-through vaginoplasty, in
which the vagina is detached from the proximal urethra and exteriorized to
the perineum, using appropriately fashioned flaps. In many cases the phallus
is too large to be recessed and is better managed by partial resection of the
corpora to recess the glans.

An IVP should be obtained if there are any urologic symptoms consistent with infection or obstructive uropathy, or if there is a family history of urologic malformations. Otherwise, an IVP is inadvisable, even though some lesions probably will be overlooked.

Bilateral cryptorchidism, on the other hand, may indicate a serious underlying problem that calls for prompt, careful inspection and, possibly, sophisticated laboratory investigation. More than 6% of patients with bilateral cryptorchidism have endocrine disorders, e.g., pituitary deficiency or primary testicular defects that cause hypogonadism.[6] A newborn "male" with hypospadias and apparent bilateral cryptorchidism may, in fact, be a virilized female who has adrenogenital syndrome (Fig 11–1). It is important to recognize this possibility early because many of these infants experience severe salt-losing adrenal cortical hyperplasia, which produces an adrenal crisis when the child is about one week old. Prompt identification is vital to effective treatment and correct gender assignment.

CHROMOSOME AND ENDOCRINE DISORDERS

Certain conditions that may be associated with cryptorchidism are given below.

KLINEFELTER'S SYNDROME. – These patients classically have gynecomastia, eunuchoidism, azospermia, small testes, hyalinization of seminiferous tubules, and elevated plasma levels of LH and FSH.[7] Most but not all such patients are chromatin positive (XXY), although they have a phenotypic male appearance (Fig 11–2). Of 93 boys operated on for cryptorchidism, three had Klinefelter's syndrome, two hypogonadotropic hypogonadism, and one germinal cell aplasia.[8]

NOONAN'S SYNDROME. – Sometimes referred to as "male Turner's syndrome," this can include cryptorchidism.[9] The distinctive facies consists of a broad forehead and hypertelorism; a flat nasal bridge; thick, low-set ears; congenital heart disease; wide-set nipples; chest wall deformity; abnormal dermatoglyphics; and cryptorchidism. These children have a normal 46 XY karyotype, and the mode of inheritance is autosomal dominant.

THE PRADER-WILLI SYNDROME. – This syndrome combines cryptorchidism, hypotonia, mental retardation, and obesity, together with dwarfism and diabetes.[10, 11] These children also have distinctive facies, so that as a group they look remarkably alike.

There are other pediatric syndromes[12, 13] that include cryptorchi-

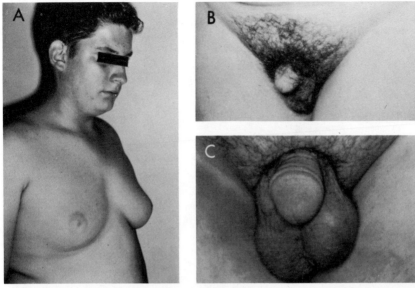

Fig 11–2.—Patient with Klinefelter's syndrome. **A,** at age 18 years prior to subareolar mastectomies. **B,** Empty scrotum. Patient had been explored at another hospital where no significant testicular tissue was found. **C,** after insertion of Silastic gel testicular prostheses to give scrotum a more normal appearance. This proved to be psychologically valuable.

dism. Although surgeons are not expected to recognize all endocrinopathies and pediatric syndromes, suffice it to say that an unusual looking child with cryptorchidism should suggest the need of prompt pediatric endocrinologic consultation. Cryptorchidism is seen in various chromosomal disorders, including Down's syndrome,[14] although a recent study of 13 cryptorchid patients at the Mayo Clinic showed no significant chromosomal abnormality.[15]

Intersexuality

At Johns Hopkins Hospital the incidence of intersexuality was 53% in 45 patients with cryptorchidism and hypospadias, including those with ambiguous genitalia.[16] Excluding patients with ambiguous genitalia, the incidence of intersexuality was 27%. Intersexuality was defined as an abnormality in (1) genetic sex (sex chromosomal aberrations such as XO/XY mosaicism), (2) gonadal sex (ovotestis or streak gonad), and (3) phenotypic sex (female or male pseudohermaphroditism), the last being the predominant disorder, seen in 10 patients. Four patients had mixed gonadal dysgenesis, and two had true

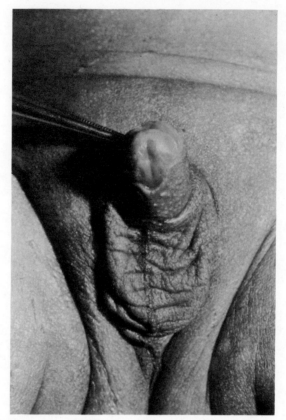

Fig 11–3.—Vanishing testis syndrome. Infant was referred with minimal degree of hypospadias, no chordee, but an empty scrotum. No gonads were palpable. Chromosome karyotype was 46 XY. There was negligible rise of plasma testosterone after five days of intramuscular administration of HCG, 1,000 units per day. Plasma gonadotropin levels were elevated. At exploration, on each side spermatic vessels ended in small nubbin of yellow gritty tissue; vas did not join this tissue. Histologic examination showed (1) primitive tubular structures that had undergone coagulation necrosis, and (2) old hemorrhage indicated by abundant hemosiderin deposits. This was testicular infarction, possibly from torsion, at 15–16 weeks of gestation.

The presence of bilateral undescended testes together with genital ambiguity should prompt thorough endocrine and anatomical investigation in the newborn period to establish the clinical problem fully. In some cases it can determine the better gender selection for the infant.

hermaphroditism and female pseudohermaphroditism, respectively. One had gonadal agenesis. Intersexuality occurred more than twice as often in patients with bilateral cryptorchidism as in those with unilateral undescent. Of the 22 patients with normal male phenotype, six intersex patients included two with mixed gonadal dysgenesis, two with male pseudohermaphroditism, one with true hermaphroditism, and one with gonadal agenesis (Fig 11–3).

ADRENOGENITAL SYNDROME. – This has been the most common intersex condition in our experience.[17] Although some of these infants have a remarkable degree of genital masculinization, they are females with normal ovaries. Nevertheless, it is not surprising that they can be mistaken for male infants with undescended testes. In some the phallus looks like a hypospadiac penis, and in rare cases it can appear totally masculine, resembling a normal penis with a phallic urethra[18-20] (see Fig 11–1). Infants with salt-losing metabolic tendency will have an adrenal crisis if not treated. In some who lack metabolic problems, however, the true nature of the child's anomaly is not appreciated until she is seen at an older age for orchiopexy or hypospadias repair. One patient, previously thought to be a male, came to our clinical attention for "hematuria," which actually was the onset of menses.

FEMINIZING TESTIS SYNDROME. – This is an especially interesting type of undescended testis seen in male pseudohermaphrodites. They are genetic males by karyotype with female-appearing genital structures. The problem may be discovered during inguinal herniorrhaphy, when a testis is found in the hernia sac, or at an older age during evaluation for infertility. The testes lie intra-abdominally or in the inguinal canal. Androgen action is deficient because of failure to bind testosterone or DHT to the nucleus (nuclear or androgen-binding protein deficiency).[21-24] This syndrome has been called familial male pseudohermaphroditism, type I; undescended testis also may occur in the same syndrome, type II, from a deficiency of the enzyme 5α-reductase, which converts testosterone to DHT.

MIXED GONADAL DYSGENESIS. – In this, the second most common intersex disorder in our experience, the genitalia may vary in appearance, one gonad often being found in the scrotum, whereas the other is not palpable, suggesting an undescended testis[25] (Fig 11–4). Characteristic gonadal findings include a dysgenic testis on one side and a streak ovary on the other. Such children should be reared as females, after alteration of the genitalia appropriately and removal of the gonads, which are at high risk of later neoplastic degeneration.

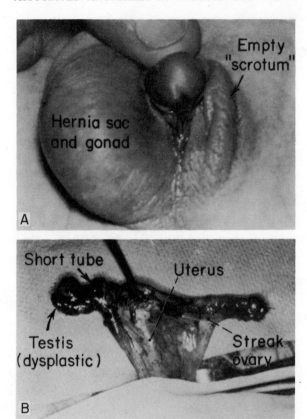

Fig 11–4.—Mixed gonadal dysgenesis, second most common type of ambiguous genitalia in the newborn infant. **A,** appearance as severe hypospadias and unilateral undescended testis. **B,** internal findings at laparotomy showing typical anatomy. On right is dysplastic testis adjacent to short fallopian tubelike structure; on left is streak ovary. There is a soft midline uterus.

True hermaphroditism. — This is one of the rarest types of ambiguous genitalia.[26] Both testicular and ovarian tissue are found in these patients. Like those with any intersex disorder, their presenting problem may be cryptorchidism combined with other genital abnormalities.

Prune Belly Syndrome

Bilateral cryptorchidism nearly always is one feature in the so-called prune belly syndrome,[27-31] a condition occurring almost exclusively in males and consisting of hypoplasia of the abdominal wall musculature and multiple severe anomalies of the urinary tract. Frequently the kidneys are dysplastic. The ureters tend to be elongated and tortuous, and massive vesicoureteral reflux usually is apparent. The bladder often is large and thick walled but not trabeculated, and there is a characteristic heart-shaped proximal urethra. In some patients the penile urethra is wide and the corpus spongiosum is absent. The skin of the abdominal wall usually is wrinkled, with the appearance of a dried prune (Fig 11–5). In a variant called "pseudo prunes" the urinary tract has the features of a full-blown case, but the abdominal wall musculature is better developed. The testes lie intra-abdominally, where normal ovaries would be in females, and tend to be underdeveloped. Standard orchiopexy is impossible in an older boy with prune belly syndrome because, despite liberal mobilization of the vessels and vas, the vessels are too short to bring the testes down into the scrotum. Therefore, in such cases we have used the approach, suggested by Fowler and Stephens,[32] of dividing the spermatic vessels and bringing the testis down on a pedicle of the vas deferens and a strip of adjacent pelvic peritoneum. The vas often is tortuous, with a beaded appearance, and the collateral blood supply to the tissues around the vas and pelvic peritoneum in these patients usually is abundant.

When we perform reconstructive surgery of the urinary tract in young infants with prune belly syndrome,[33] we do an orchiopexy at the same time. In children of this age, we have found it possible to gain sufficient length to bring the testes into the scrotum without dividing the vessels. The apparent reason for this is that the distance the testis must be moved becomes greater as the patient grows older. Small infants are short and wide but, with maturation, their geometry changes, elongating and narrowing so that the distance to the scrotum becomes relatively longer.

ABNORMALITIES OF PARATESTICULAR STRUCTURES

Normal genital development in the male requires müllerian inhibiting substance. This material is elaborated by the primitive gonad, causing regression of the müllerian duct structures, and by androgen, which is required for maturation of the wolffian duct into epididymis, vas deferens, and seminal vesicles.[34, 35] Already cited has been Hunter's conjecture whether an undescended testis was abnormal because it failed to descend, or whether it failed to descend because it was abnormal.[36] It may be that failure to descend results from inadequate

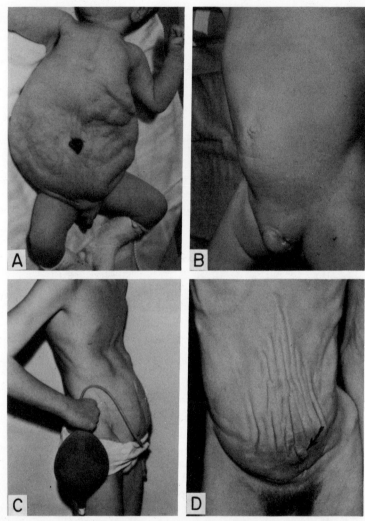

Fig 11–5.—Prune belly syndrome with intra-abdominal undescended testes. **A,** severe neonatal case with wrinkling of abdominal wall. Note visible loops of bowel and ureters through hypoplastic abdominal wall, especially on left. (Casts were put on clubbed feet.) **B,** eight-week-old infant with slight wrinkling of skin of lower abdomen, somewhat better abdominal wall musculature than in **(A)** but typical internal findings of prune belly syndrome. **C,** 13-year-old boy with less obvious wrinkling but protuberant lower abdomen and pectus excavatum. Long-standing cystostomy. **D,** 15-year-old boy with severe abdominal wall wrinkling. Note end ureterostomies *(arrow).* The two infants **(A** and **B)** underwent primary reconstructive urologic surgery

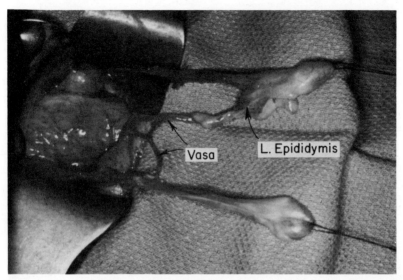

Fig 11–6.—Abnormal vas and epididymis. Patient had multiple anomalies including esophageal atresia, malrotation, duodenal stenosis, and imperforate anus, all corrected at birth. Bilateral orchiopexy was performed at age 10 months. Although both testes were intra-abdominal, mobilization provided sufficient length to place them in scrotum without tension. This usually is impossible with high cryptorchids in whom operation is delayed until an older age. Left testis shows attenuated epididymis joined by vas. Right testis shows absence of epididymis, and vas ends blindly about 3 cm proximal to testis.

hormone activity, causing the gubernaculum to shorten.[37] It is probable in many cases that the undescended testis was abnormal from the outset, and thus not surprising that there is a comparatively high incidence of associated abnormalities in structures developing from the wolffian duct (Figs 11–6 and 11–7). In a review of 168 boys with undescended testes, Waaler[38] noted malformations or absence of the epididymis in 3.6% and disruption of the vas or epididymis in 3.3%. Marshall and Shermeta[39] prepared a prospective study of the paratesticular anatomy of 42 undescended testes in 38 boys, and found 36% with an abnormality, commonly an elongated looplike epididymis. These

and orchiopexy. The two older boys (**C** and **D**) underwent undiversion operations, i.e., reconstructions with discarding of urinary diversions. Orchiopexy was done by the Fowler-Stephens technique (dividing spermatic vessels and bringing testes into scrotum on pedicle of vas and adjacent peritoneum).

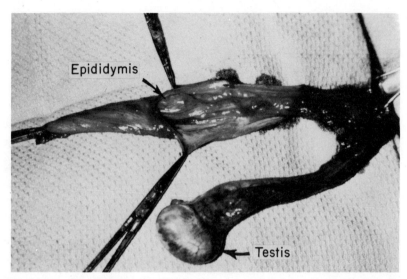

Fig 11–7.—Separation of testis from epididymis. At end of spermatic vessels is well-formed testis. Vas ended blindly in fibrous epididymis anatomically separate from testis, all lying intra-abdominally, and yet there was ample length for it to reach scrotum, which is unusual. Anorchia had been previously diagnosed mistakenly by venography, which did not show spermatic veins..Opposite side had been explored earlier and no testis found.

authors also found agenesis of the epididymis as well as atresia or loss of its continuity, making it likely that many undescended testes will be infertile despite early and adequate orchiopexy, since there is no egress for sperm. Other authors have described similar findings.[40-43] These patients may have an anomaly of the prostatic utricle[44] or even a sizable vagina communicating with the urethra, especially in bilateral cases, indicating deficiency of the müllerian inhibiting substance in utero (Fig 11–8). It has been suggested that when an abnormality of the paratesticular ducts is seen during orchiopexy, the urinary tract should be thoroughly investigated for other significant anomalies.[45]

TORSION OF THE TESTIS

Testicular torsion is likely to occur in cryptorchidism (Fig 11–9). During a 10-year period, Johnston[46] observed that the testis was undescended in 15 of 65 boys admitted to the Alder Hey Children's Hospital with torsion of the testis; nine of the 15 were under one year of age. Noting that previous reports of 430 cases of testicular torsion implicated nondescent of the testis in 54%, Johnston theorized that

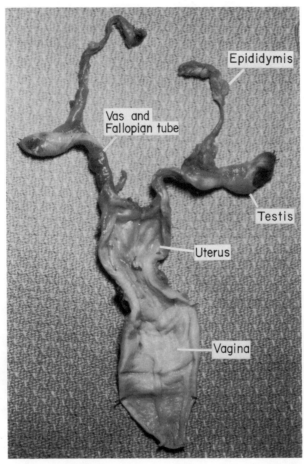

Fig 11–8.—Retained müllerian duct structures. Five-year-old boy referred for hypospadias repair and bilateral orchiopexy. Because of genital abnormality and cryptorchidism, karyotyping had been done at birth and boy was found to be 46 XY; therefore, no further investigation was performed at the time. He had peculiar facies, a broad nasal bridge, and high-arched palate, as well as bilateral syndactyly of second and third toes. Serum testosterone and gonadotropin levels were within normal limits for a child age five. Exploration revealed bilateral intra-abdominal testes. Biopsy showed small seminiferous tubules, lined with Sertoli cells and filled with microcalcifications. There were no germ cells, and Leydig cells were sparse. It was decided to remove testes together with inappropriate uterus and vagina. Hypospadias repair was carried out subsequently, and later bilateral testicular prostheses were placed in scrotum.

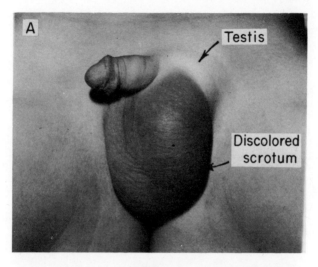

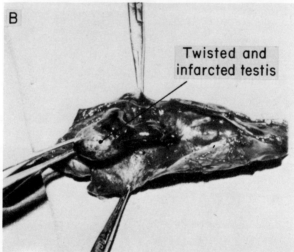

Fig 11–9.—Testicular torsion in cryptorchidism. **A,** three-year-old boy with tender swollen mass in left midgroin and scrotal redness. **B,** appearance of twisted testis at operation.

this discrepancy might reflect the more frequent use of orchiopexy today, which would prevent subsequent torsion. Leape[47] reported cryptorchidism in eight of 50 patients with testicular torsion, observing, however, that torsion of the testicular appendages is not more common in boys with undescended testis than in normal boys. In those with testicular torsion, whether or not the testis is undescended, prophylactic fixation of the opposite testis to prevent contralateral torsion is generally recommended.

INGUINAL HERNIA

Although indirect inguinal hernia is common when there is true testicular undescent,[48] if the testis is descended but ectopic it is unlikely to occur. In only a few cases is the inguinal hernia symptomatic. If a young infant has a symptomatic hernia requiring operation, not only should the hernia sac be removed but the testis should be placed down in the scrotum. We have encountered many boys with a previous inguinal hernia incision, who were referred to us for orchiopexy, whose families were told that "it will come down on its own when he grows older." In our experience this never happens; operative adhesions created during herniorrhaphy will keep the high-riding testis in the same position. Thus orchiopexy should always accompany hernia repair if the testis is not in the scrotum, no matter how young the child. Orchiopexy is accomplished easily with minimal mobilization of the cord structures in the small infant. Seldom is complete retroperitoneal mobilization of the vas and vessels necessary in infants, whereas in older boys it is almost routine. Inguinal hernia and undescended testes commonly occur in boys with exstrophy of the bladder.

MATERNAL DIETHYLSTILBESTROL ADMINISTRATION

It has been well documented that the use of diethylstilbestrol to prevent miscarriage caused adenosis and even malignancy of the vagina in daughters of some of these patients.[49] Recently, study of male offspring of such mothers showed a slightly higher than expected incidence of undescended testes,[50] as well as epididymal cysts and other genitourinary abnormalities.

WILMS' TUMOR

There is an association of Wilms' tumor with aniridia and with hemihypertrophy. Cryptorchidism also appears to be more common in boys with Wilms' tumor; in a review of 223 boys with this condition,[51] 11 had undescended testes (five unilateral, six bilateral). This is more than three times the expected frequency in the general population. Bond[52] reported 10 patients with bilateral Wilms' tumor, of whom seven had other genitourinary abnormalities, including bilateral cryptorchidism in two.

CONCLUSION

In patients with undescended testis, especially in bilateral cases, the clinician should look at the entire patient. A high index of suspicion will lead to early discovery of an associated anomaly in some patients.

REFERENCES

1. Felton L.M.: Should intravenous pyelography be a routine procedure for children with cryptorchidism or hypospadias? *J. Urol.* 81:335, 1959.
2. Grossman H., Pirie D.: The incidence of urinary tract anomalies in cryptorchid boys. *Am. J. Roentgenol.* 103:210, 1968.
3. Noe H.N., Patterson T.H.: Screening urography in asymptomatic cryptorchid patients. *J. Urol.* 119:669, 1978.
4. Watson R.A., Lennox K.W., Gangai M.P.: Simple cryptorchidism: The value of the excretory urogram as a screening method. *J. Urol.* 111:789, 1974.
5. Tveter K.J., Fjaerli J.: Roentgenological findings in cryptorchidism. *Scand. J. Urol. Nephrol.* 9:171, 1975.
6. Fonkalsrud E.W.: The undescended testis. *Curr. Probl. Surg.* 15:15, 1978.
7. Klinefelter H.F. Jr., Reifenstein E.C. Jr., Albright F.: Syndrome characterized by gynecomastia, aspermatogenesis without A-leydigism, and increased excretion of follicle-stimulating hormone. *J. Clin. Endocrinol.* 2:615, 1942.
8. Hortling H., de la Chapelle A., Johansson C.J., et al.: An endocrinologic follow-up study of operated cases of cryptorchidism. *J. Clin. Endocrinol.* 27:120, 1967.
9. Redman J.: Noonan's syndrome and cryptorchidism. *J. Urol.* 109:909, 1973.
10. Prader A., Labhart A., Willi H.: Ein Syndrom von Adipositas, Kleinwuchs, Kryptorchismus und Oligophrenie nach myatonieartigem Zustand im Neugeborenenalter. *Schweiz. Med. Wochenschr.* 86:1260, 1956.
11. Laurance B.M.: Hypotonia, mental retardation, obesity and cryptorchidism associated with dwarfism and diabetes in children. *Arch. Dis. Child,* 42:126, 1967.
12. Smith D.: *Recognizable Patterns of Human Malformations: Genetic, Embryologic and Clinical Aspects*, ed. 2. Major Problems in Clinical Pediatrics, vol. 7. Philadelphia, W.B. Saunders Co., 1976.
13. Lowe C.U., Terry M., MacLachlan E.A.: Organic aciduria, decreased renal ammonia production, hydrophthalmos and mental retardation. *Am. J. Dis. Child.* 83:164, 1952.
14. Lewandowski R.C. Jr., Yunis J.: New chromosomal syndromes. *Am. J. Dis. Child.* 129:515, 1975.
15. Dewald G.W., Kelalis P., Gordon H.: Chromosomal studies in cryptorchidism. *J. Urol.* 117:110, 1977.
16. Rajfer J., Walsh P.C.: The incidence of intersexuality in patients with hypospadias and cryptorchidism. *J. Urol.* 116:769, 1976.
17. Hendren W.H., Crawford J.D.: The child with ambiguous genitalia. *Curr. Probl. Surg.* 1:64, 1972.

18. Maxted W., Baker R., McCrystal H., et al.: Complete masculinization of the external genitalia in congenital adrenocortical hyperplasia: Presentation of two cases. *J. Urol.* 94:266, 1965.
19. Rosenberg B., Hendren W.H., Crawford J.D.: Posterior urethrovaginal communication in apparent males with congenital adrenocortical hyperplasia. *N. Engl. J. Med.* 280:131, 1969.
20. Hendren W.H., Crawford J.D.: Adrenogenital syndrome: The anatomy of the anomaly and its repair. Some new concepts. *J. Pediatr. Surg.* 4:49, 1969.
21. Donahoe P.K., Crawford J.D., Hendren W.H.: Management of neonates and children with male pseudohermaphroditism. *J. Pediatr. Surg.* 12: 1045, 1977.
22. Madden J.D., Walsh P.C., MacDonald P.C., et al.: Clinical and endocrinologic characterization of a patient with the syndrome of incomplete testicular feminization. *J. Clin. Endocrinol. Metab.* 41:751, 1975.
23. Wilson J.D., Harrod M.J., Goldstein J.L., et al.: Familial incomplete male pseudohermaphroditism, type I. *N. Engl. J. Med.* 290:1097, 1974.
24. Walsh P.C., Madden J.D., Harrod M.J., et al.: Familial incomplete male pseudohermaphroditism, type II. *N. Engl. J. Med.* 291:944, 1974.
25. Donahoe P.K., Crawford J.D., Hendren W.H.: Mixed gonadal dysgenesis, pathogenesis and management. *J. Pediatr. Surg.* 14:287, 1979.
26. Donahoe P.K., Crawford J.D., Hendren W.H.: True hermaphroditism: A clinical description and a proposed function for the long arm of the Y chromosome. *J. Pediatr. Surg.* 13:293, 1978.
27. Eagle J.F. Jr., Barret G.S.: Congenital deficiency of abdominal musculature with associated genitourinary abnormalities: A syndrome. *Pediatrics* 6:721, 1950.
28. Silverman F.N., Huang N.: Congenital absence of the abdominal muscles associated with malformation of the genitourinary and alimentary tracts. *Am. J. Dis. Child.* 80:91, 1950.
29. Lattimer J.K.: Congenital deficiency of the abdominal musculature and associated genitourinary anomalies: A report of 22 cases. *J. Urol.* 79:313, 1958.
30. Welch K.J., Kearney G.P.: Abdominal musculature deficiency syndrome: Prune belly. *J. Urol.* 111:693, 1974.
31. Hendren W.H.: Prune belly syndrome, in Devine C.J. Jr., Stecker J.F. Jr. (eds.): *Textbook of Urology.* Boston, Little, Brown & Co., 1978.
32. Fowler R., Stephens F.D.: The role of testicular vascular anatomy in the salvage of high undescended testis. *Aust. N.Z. J. Surg.* 29:92, 1959.
33. Hendren W.H.: A new approach to the infant with severe obstructive uropathy: Early complete reconstruction. *J. Pediatr. Surg.* 5:184, 1970.
34. Donahoe P.K., Ito Y., Morikawa Y., et al.: Müllerian inhibiting substance in human testes after birth. *J. Pediatr. Surg.* 12:323, 1977.
35. Federman D.D.: *Abnormal Sexual Development: A Genetic and Endocrine Approach to Differential Diagnosis.* Philadelphia, W.B. Saunders Co., 1967.
36. Hunter J.: Observations on the state of the testis in the foetus and on the hernia congenita, *in Medical Commentaries*, part I. London, A. Hamilton, 1762, p. 75.

37. Radhakrishnan J., Morikawa Y., Donahoe P.K., et al.: Observations on the gubernaculum during descent of the testis. *Invest. Urol.* 16:365, 1979.
38. Waaler P.E.: Clinical and cytogenetic studies in undescended testes. *Acta Paediatr. Scand.* 65:553, 1976.
39. Marshall F.F., Shermeta D.W.: Epididymal abnormalities associated with undescended testis. *J. Urol.* 121:341, 1979.
40. Dean A.L., Major J.W., Ottenheimer E.J.: Failure of fusion of the testis and epididymis. *J. Urol.* 68:754, 1952.
41. Mahour G.H., Woolley M.M.: Failure of urogenital union. *J. Pediatr. Surg.* 7:442, 1972.
42. Dickinson S.J.: Structural abnormalities in the undescended testis. *J. Pediatr. Surg.* 8:523, 1973.
43. Davis E.L., Shpall R.A., Goldstein A.M.B., et al.: Congenitally uncoiled epididymis in a cryptorchid testicle. *J. Urol.* 111:618, 1974.
44. Workman C., Porch P., Rhamy R.K.: The congenitally dilated prostatic utricle. *J. Urol.* 120:508, 1978.
45. Bishop M.C., Whitaker R.H., Sherwood T.: Associated renal anomalies in familial cryptorchidism. *Lancet* 2:249, 1979.
46. Johnston J.H.: The undescended testis. *Arch. Dis. Child.* 40:113, 1965.
47. Leape L.: Torsion of the testis: Invitation to error. *J.A.M.A.* 200:669, 1967.
48. Gross R.E., Jewett T.C. Jr.: Surgical experiences from 1222 operations for undescended testis. *J.A.M.A.* 160:634, 1956.
49. Herbst A.L., Ulfelder H., Poskanzer D.C.: Adenocarcinoma of the vagina: Association of maternal stilbestrol therapy with tumor appearance in young women. *N. Engl. J. Med.* 284:878, 1971.
50. Cosgrove M.D., Benton B., Henderson B.E.: Male genitourinary abnormalities and maternal diethylstilbestrol. *J. Urol.* 117:220, 1977.
51. Miller R.W., Fraumeni J.F. Jr., Manning M.D.: Association of Wilms' tumor with aniridia, hemihypertrophy, and other congenital malformations. *N. Engl. J. Med.* 270:922, 1964.
52. Bond J.V.: Bilateral Wilms' tumor and urinary tract anomalies. *Lancet* 2: 721, 1975.

12 / Genetic and Endocrinologic Syndromes Associated with Cryptorchidism

MITCHELL E. GEFFNER, M.D.
BARBARA M. LIPPE, M.D.

AS AN ISOLATED ABNORMALITY, cryptorchidism occurs in 0.8–1.8% of male babies when examined at one year of age.[1, 2] With the concomitant presence of dysmorphological features, this incidence increases significantly. Similarly over 6% of males with bilateral cryptorchidism have associated endocrinologic disorders, including idiopathic or genetic hypopituitarism, idiopathic hypogonadotropic hypogonadism, familial hypogonadism (Kallman's syndrome), or primary testicular defects.[3] In addition, bilateral cryptorchidism is a component of several anomalads involving the abdominal wall, including abdominal muscle deficiency (the Eagle-Barrett prune belly syndrome), exstrophy of the bladder, or presence of a cloaca, and occurs commonly in infants with gastroschisis and omphalocele[4] (see Chapter 11). Furthermore, bilateral cryptorchidism is associated with an increased incidence of both major and minor renal anomalies,[5] hypospadias, and ipsilateral abnormalities of the epididymis and vas deferens.[4] Finally, cryptorchidism is a variable feature of many complex human malformation syndromes. Table 12–1 lists conditions in which cryptorchidism occurs with greater than expected frequency. We have chosen to group these according to the following categories: chromosomal defects, syndromes with known inheritance patterns, syndromes with probable or possible genetic significance, disorders acquired in utero, and endocrine disorders.

CHROMOSOMAL

Although cryptorchidism is a very frequent component of syndromes associated with extra or deleted autosomal material (see Table

TABLE 12-1. — SYNDROMES ASSOCIATED
WITH CRYPTORCHIDISM

SYNDROME	FREQUENCY OF SYNDROME°	FREQUENCY OF CRYPTORCHIDISM‡
Chromosomal		
Autosomal		
Trisomy 8	CR†	+
Trisomy 13	1/5,000	+++
Trisomy 18 (Edwards)	0.3/1,000	+++
Trisomy 21 (Down's)	1/660	+
Triploidy	CR	++
4p- (Wolf-Hirschhorn)	CR	++
5p- (Cri-du-chat)	CR	+
13q-	CR	++
18q-	CR	++
21q-	CR	+
Sexual		
XYY	1/840 males	+
XXY (Klinefelter)	1/450 males	+
XXXXY	CR	+
Autosomal dominant§		
Basal cell nevus	CR	+
Opitz	CR	++
Popliteal web	CR	+
Saethre-Chotzen	CR	+
Steinert myotonic dystrophy	CR	+
Treacher-Collins	CR	+
Autosomal recessive§		
Cockayne	CR	++
Cryptophthalmos	CR	++
Dubowitz	CR	++
Diastrophic dwarfism	CR	+
Ellis-van Creveld	CR	+
Fanconi pancytopenia	CR	+
Meckel-Gruber	CR	++
Roberts	CR	++
Robinow	CR	+
Seckel	CR	+
Smith-Lemli-Opitz	CR	++
Zellweger (cerebrohepatorenal)	CR	+
X-linked§		
Aarskog (facial-digital-genital)	CR	++
Lowe (oculocerebrorenal)	CR	++
Sporadic‖		
Beckwith-Wiedemann	CR	+
Coffin-Siris	CR	+
Cornelia de Lange	CR	++
Femoral hypoplasia — unusual facies	CR	+
Gorlin fronto-metaphyseal hypoplasia	CR	+
Hallerman-Streiff	CR	+
Noonan	1/1,000	++

(continued)

TABLE 12-1.—SYNDROMES ASSOCIATED
WITH CRYPTORCHIDISM (CONT.)

SYNDROME	FREQUENCY OF SYNDROME°	FREQUENCY OF CRYPTORCHIDISM‡
Prader-Willi	CR	+ +
Rubinstein-Taybi	CR	+ +
Anomalads‖		
Abdominal muscle deficiency		
(prune belly)		
Exstrophy of the bladder		
Exstrophy of the cloaca		
Acquired¶		
Congenital rubella		+
Fetal hydantoin		+
Endocrine		
Hypothalamic-pituitary		
Intersexuality		
Testicular enzymatic		
Testicular cellular		

°Frequencies taken from Smith,[6] Bergsma,[7] or Rimoin and Schimke.[8]
†CR = case reports
‡+++ = occurs in 100% of cases; ++ = occurs in 50-99% of cases; + = occurs in less than 50% of cases.
§Known inheritance pattern.
‖Probable or possible genetic significance.
¶Acquired in utero.

12-1), such conditions themselves are relatively rare and often lethal, except for trisomy 21 (Down's syndrome). Thus, the pediatrician or surgeon seeing a cryptorchid patient with multiple associated phenotypic features should recognize the possibility of the chromosomal defect if not already identified. Even in the newborn period, infants with trisomy 21 may have characteristic facies with macroglossia, a small nose with low nasal bridge, hypertelorism, slanted palpebral fissures (mongoloid slant), and epicanthal folds. Other variable findings include simian crease; fifth finger anomalies and wide gaps between the first and second toes; cardiac anomalies, most commonly atrioventricular canal defects; and neurologic deficits, including hypotonia and microcephaly. The incidence of cryptorchidism in trisomy 21 ranges from 14% to 27% depending on the age at diagnosis. As a rule, such patients also are hypogonadal or at least appear to be of low fertility.[6]

Both trisomy 18 (Edwards' syndrome) and trisomy 13, although much less common than Down's syndrome, are associated with undescended testes in 100% of males. Trisomy 18 patients traditionally have clenched hands, short sternums, and low arch-dermal ridge patterning on their fingertips, as well as a myriad of other skeletal, CNS, and cardiovascular anomalies. Often associated with pre- and postnatal growth deficiency, 90% of these affected infants die within the first year,[6] usually from pulmonary complications. Children with trisomy 13 classically demonstrate holoprosencephalic defects with variable degrees of incomplete forebrain development as well as defects of optic and olfactory nerves, severe mental deficiency, cleft lip and/or palate, parieto-occipital scalp defects, polydactyly, hyperconvex fingernails, and prominent heels (rocker-bottom feet). Only 18% of affected infants survive beyond the first year of life.[6] Because of the excessive infant mortality associated with both trisomy 18 and 13, the question of surgical repair of nonlethal genitourinary anomalies, including cryptorchidism, should be postponed until after the first few months so that the issue of survival is decided.

Of the sex chromosomal aberrations (see Table 12–1) associated with genital abnormalities in the phenotypic male, Klinefelter's syndrome (classically 46 XXY) is the prototype. Occurring in about one of every 450 males, Klinefelter's syndrome is most frequently associated with hypogonadism, as manifest by small postpubertal testes concomitant with the histologic picture of hyalinization and fibrosis of seminiferous tubules and loss of germinal epithelium with Leydig cell hyperplasia.[9] What was originally believed to be a high incidence of cryptorchidism in this disorder probably reflects an increased frequency of small, easily retractile testes. Nevertheless, Laron[10] and Bergada et al.[11] still hold that a somewhat higher than normal proportion of undescended testes exists in patients with Klinefelter's syndrome. Of importance from a surgical standpoint is that affected males with mosaic karyotypes (e.g., 46 XY/ 47 XXY) have less severe testicular damage[12] and may in fact have the potential for fertility.[13] Thus appropriately timed orchiopexy in the cryptorchid male with a mosaic Klinefelter karyotype may enhance his ultimate potential for spermatogenesis and therefore is an appropriate consideration. In the 47 XXY male, orchiopexy is intended primarily for extra-abdominal placement of the gonad to facilitate examination, and the timing will not enhance fertility, which is virtually zero.

AUTOSOMAL DOMINANT, RECESSIVE, AND X-LINKED

Referring again to Table 12–1, it may be seen that cryptorchidism is a relatively minor feature of syndromes inherited in either an autosomal dominant or autosomal recessive pattern. Of the conditions inherited in an X-linked fashion, the Aarskog facial-digital-genital syndrome, although extremely rare, bears mentioning. Of the approximately 50 reported affected males, 70% have had cryptorchidism and greater than 90% have a shawl or saddle scrotum in which the scrotal folds extend around the ventral surface of the penis, resembling fused labia majora. However, fertility has been documented with either defect, so that orchiopexy is indicated.[14]

SPORADIC

Of the so-called sporadic conditions in which cryptorchidism may be a common occurrence, two syndromes are representative (see Table 12-1). The first is Noonan's syndrome, which may occur as frequently as one in 1,000 births.[7] Previously described as male Turner's syndrome because of a similar phenotype, this condition is now known to occur in both males and females and is totally unrelated to Turner's syndrome. Characteristic features of Noonan's syndrome include a high incidence of mild mental retardation; abnormal facies with epicanthal folds, hypertelorism, and ptosis; congenital defects of the right side of the heart, most commonly pulmonic stenosis; and short stature. In addition, of the males with Noonan's syndrome, 70% will have cryptorchidism.[7] Puberty, although often delayed, does occur spontaneously, so that timed orchiopexy is indicated.[15]

The second important sporadic condition associated with cryptorchidism is the Prader-Willi syndrome. More than 200 cases have been described.[6] Such patients typically manifest intrauterine and neonatal hypotonia, feeding problems, and delayed milestones; later they usually are significantly mentally retarded and are short and obese. Cryptorchidism occurs in 84% of affected males. However, in both sexes there is a high incidence of hypogonadism, which is secondary to central hypogonadotropism rather than being of testicular or ovarian origin. Thus orchiopexy, although indicated at some time to bring down the testes, usually does not alter the potential for fertility. Additionally, such patients usually will have progressive, severe personality problems, often requiring institutionalization.[16]

ACQUIRED

Finally, bilateral undescended testes have been noted in several conditions acquired in utero of either an infectious (congenital rubella) or teratogenic nature (fetal hydantoin syndrome). Details of the clinical features of these syndromes, as well as all others mentioned in Table 12-1, are given in excellent review texts by Smith[6] and Rimoin and Schimke.[8]

ENDOCRINE

Bilateral cryptorchidism, as a consequence of primary endocrinologic disorders, may occur with hypothalamic-pituitary dysfunction, sex chromosomal mosaicism associated with ambiguous genitalia, and primary testicular defects (see Table 12–1). The common link in disorders of the hypothalamic-pituitary axis appears to be hypogonadotropism, as undescended testes can occur in panhypopituitarism, hypogonadotropic hypogonadism, and Kallman's syndrome (sex-limited anosmia and/or midline facial defects with isolated gonadotropin defects). However, multiple studies reviewed in Chapter 8 conclude that even bilateral cryptorchidism is a heterogeneous condition that, in some patients, appears related to central dysfunction and, in others, is primarily of testicular origin. The significance of recognizing a central gonadotropin-deficient cause for the cryptorchidism, however, is twofold: (1) if associated pituitary hormones are deficient, the deficits may be treatable with replacement hormone therapy; and (2) the availability of both HCG-HMG and LH-RH (an intranasal preparation for long-term use currently under FDA phase 2 study) allows treatment of the hypogonadism by direct stimulation of the testis. Thus fertility as well as androgenization is possible, and timed orchiopexy is therefore indicated.

In a study of 75 patients with hypopituitarism beginning in childhood, Brasel et al.[17] noted that 45 (60%) had isolated growth hormone deficiency or additional trophic hormone deficiencies on an idiopathic basis; 19 (25%) had organic hypopituitarism secondary to CNS lesions, most commonly craniopharyngioma; and 11 (15%) had isolated gonadotropin deficiency.[17] The male with nonorganic gonadotropin deficiency usually is characterized by sexual infantilism, which may manifest as micropenis, an underdeveloped scrotum, and/or cryptorchidism.[18] When associated with growth hormone deficiency, short stature usually is seen between 12 and 18 months of age. However, if accurate growth records are available, slow growth may be detected within the first year of life. Additionally, the biochemical consequences of hypopituitarism may manifest in early infancy as hypoglycemic convulsions. In fact, the combination of hypoglycemia and microgenitalia in a male infant points strongly toward hypopituitarism. Physical characteristics of affected children who show the hypopituitarism later in childhood are variable. Aside from the aforementioned genital abnormalities, these patients usually are mildly overweight for their height, with excess fat accumulation usually overlying the abdomen and the cheeks. This cherubic appearance reflects a deficiency of antilipolysis normally stimulated by growth hormone. Organic causes of hypothalamic-pituitary insufficiency often are seen in later childhood with combinations of endocrine, visual, and neurologic signs and symptoms. Cryptorchidism usually is not a consequence of these acquired lesions, although pubertal delay and sexual infantilism are common.

Awareness of midline neurofacial defects associated with hypothalamic-pituitary deficiency has increased over the past 10 years. Although signs may be obvious, as in the holoprosencephalies, other related conditions may manifest subtle clinical findings, so that some may have originally been categorized in the idiopathic group.[17] Thus almost 50% of patients with hypopituitarism may have an anatomical lesion. The prototype midline defect is the cleft lip or palate. Children with isolated cleft lip or palate are growth hormone deficient about 40 times more often than are unaffected children;[19] they also may have other trophic hormone deficiencies. This association may result from the embryologic relation of the adenohypophysis and oral ectoderm. Thus the child with a midline cleft, short stature, and microgenitalia or cryptorchidism must not be classified as having multiple congenital anomalies. Instead the cryptorchidism may be part of the hypopituitarism and timed surgical repair is indicated, since exogenous administration of gonadotropic hormones may stimulate testicular development and result in the potential for fertility. A similar approach should be directed toward the child with midline hypopituitarism associated with septo-optic dysplasia (unilateral or bilateral optic nerve hypoplasia with amblyopia and searching nystagmus; absent septum pellucidum in about 50% of cases; and variable trophic hormone insufficiencies)[20] or a single unpaired maxillary central incisor (either deciduous or permanent), if cryptorchidism is present.[21]

Hypogonadotropic hypogonadism with anosmia as described by Kallman in 1944 also was variably characterized by gynecomastia and abnormalities of color vision.[22] In addition, Bardin et al.[23] have noted the occurrence of inguinal or abdominal testes in four of seven affected patients. Furthermore, unpublished observations by McPherson have noted the association of true anorchism and hypogonadotropism with anosmia.[24] Thus in older cryptorchid children, testing of olfactory activity should not be overlooked. Identification of such patients is important in that gonadal responsiveness with subsequent fertility may occur after long-term administration of HCG-HMG or LH-RH.

The newborn infant with ambiguous genitalia and bilaterally undescended testes (intersexuality) mandates an immediate and thorough evaluation to guarantee proper gender assignment and sex of rearing. Such a clinical presentation may represent any of the intersex anomalies including male pseudohermaphroditism, true hermaphroditism, asymmetric gonadal dysgenesis, or female virilization most commonly associated with congenital adrenal hyperplasia (21-hydroxylase deficiency). This situation constitutes a medical and/or surgical emergency and requires the urgent cooperation of pediatrician, endocrinologist, geneticist, radiologist, and surgeon (see Chapter 11).

Finally, primary testicular defects (see Table 12–1) that may be associated with cryptorchidism include enzymatic defects in testosterone synthesis, disorders of androgen end-organ insensitivity, and Sertoli cell-only syndrome. In these situations, cryptorchidism usually is an uncommon occurrence, ambiguous genitalia and/or infertility being much more prominent features. However, recognition of the association is important, since orchiopexy, although indicated for gonadal placement, may not improve pubertal masculinization or fertility.

REFERENCES

1. Scorer C.G.: The incidence of incomplete descent of the testicle at birth. *Arch. Dis. Child.* 31:198, 1956.
2. Buemann B., Henriksen H., Villumsen A.L., et al.: Incidence of undescended testis in the newborn. *Acta Chir. Scand.* [Suppl.] 283:289, 1961.
3. Hortling H., de la Chappelle A., Johansson C.J., et al.: An endocrinologic follow-up study of operated cases of cryptorchidism. *J. Clin. Endocrinol. Metab.* 27:120, 1967.
4. Fonkalsrud E.W.: The undescended testis. *Curr. Probl. Surg.* 15:1, 1978.
5. Cook G.T., Marshall V.F.: The association of undescended testes and renal abnormalities. Presented at annual meeting of American Academy of Pediatrics, Washington, D.C., Nov. 1968.
6. Smith D.W.: *Recognizable Patterns of Human Malformation.* Philadelphia, W.B. Saunders Co., 1976.
7. Bergsma D.: *Birth Defects Atlas and Compendium.* Baltimore, Williams & Wilkins Co., 1973.
8. Rimoin D.L., Schimke R.N.: *Genetic Disorders of the Endocrine Glands.* St. Louis, C.V. Mosby Co., 1971.
9. Paulsen C.A.: The testis, in Williams R.H. (ed.): *Textbook of Endocrinology.* Philadelphia, W.B. Saunders Co., 1968.
10. Laron Z.: Klinefelter's syndrome: Early diagnosis and social aspects. *Hosp. Pract.* 7:135, 1972.
11. Bergada C., Farias N.E., Romero de Behar B.M., et al.: Abnormal sex chromatin pattern in cryptorchidism, girls with short stature and other endocrine patients. *Helv. Paediatr. Acta* 24:372, 1969.
12. Gordon D.L., Kampotic E., Thomas W., et al.: Pathologic testicular findings in Klinefelter's syndrome. *Arch. Intern. Med.* 130:726, 1972.
13. Warburg E.: A fertile patient with Klinefelter's syndrome. *Acta Endocrinol.* 43:12, 1963.

14. Sugarman G.I., Rimoin D.L., Lachman R.S.: The facio-digital-genital (Aarskog) syndrome. *Am. J. Dis. Child.* 126:248, 1973.
15. Saez J.M., Morera A.M., Bertrand J.: Testicular endocrine function in males with Noonan's syndrome. *Lancet* 2:1078, 1969.
16. Hall B.D., Smith D.W.: Prader-Willi syndrome. *J. Pediatr.* 81:286, 1972.
17. Brasel J.A., Wright J.C., Wilkins L., et al.: An evaluation of seventy-five patients with hypopituitarism beginning in childhood. *Am. J. Med.* 38:484, 1963.
18. Frasier S.D.: Growth disorders in children. *Ped. Clin. North Am.* 26:1, 1979.
19. Rudman D., Davis G.T., Priest J.H.: Prevalence of growth hormone deficiency in children with cleft lip or palate. *J. Pediatr.* 93:378, 1978.
20. Patel H., Tze W.J., Crichton J.U., et al.: Optic nerve hypoplasia with hypopituitarism. *Am. J. Dis. Child.* 129:175, 1975.
21. Rappaport E.B., Ulstrom R.A., Gorlin R.J., et al.: Solitary maxillary central incisor and short stature. *J. Pediatr.* 91:924, 1977.
22. Kallmann F.J., Schoenfeld W.A., Barrera, S.E.: The genetic aspects of primary eunuchoidism. *Am. J. Ment. Defic.* 48:203, 1944.
23. Bardin C.W., Ross G.T., Rifkind A.B., et al.: Studies of the pituitary-Leydig cell axis in young men with hypogonadotropic hypogonadism and hypospermia: Comparison with normal men, prepubertal boys, and hypopituitary patients. *J. Clin. Invest.* 48:2046, 1969.
24. Males J.L., Townsend J.L., Schneider R.A.: Hypogonadotrophic hypogonadism with anosmia — Kallman's syndrome. *Arch. Intern. Med.* 131:501, 1973.

13 / Malignancy and the Undescended Testis

DONALD C. MARTIN, M.D.

THE RELATIONSHIP between cryptorchidism and germinal cell tumors of the testis, long a concern to physicians, has received increased emphasis in the medical literature in recent years. LeConte in 1851 is credited with being the first to focus attention on the tumor potential of the undescended testis.[1] Despite numerous reports dealing with this association during the past century, on the basis of their experience some surgeons deny that the relationship is significant.[2, 3] Because cryptorchidism is uncommon and only a small proportion of patients with the anomaly subsequently will have malignancy, it is not surprising that some senior surgeons have never encountered a case. However, the experience of others differs, substantiating the more widely held tumorigenic relationship. Green et al.[4] collected 20 cases from the records of two university hospitals in a survey during a 10-year span.

INCIDENCE

Reports summarizing large series of patients with testicular tumors include many whose germinal cell tumors developed from antecedent cryptorchid testes (Table 13–1). This association has varied from 3.5% to 12.9%, with a mean of about 10%.[5-8] As indicated, 9.8% of all germinal cell tumors arise in cryptorchid testes, a fact that is startling to most physicians and unbelievable to some surgeons.

The increased danger of development of a malignancy can be determined if the population at risk is defined. Campbell[5] extensively surveyed the incidence of cryptorchidism in young recruits in the armies of Europe and America and found a 0.28% incidence. His review spanned most of the 100 years from the mid-19th to the mid-20th centuries. If we accept Campbell's incidence of 0.28%, a multiple of 35 would be required to raise this small population at risk to the ob-

TABLE 13-1.—INCIDENCE OF CRYPTORCHIDISM AMONG TESTICULAR
TUMORS AND INCREASED HAZARD TO CRYPTORCHID PATIENT°

SERIES	NO. OF PTS. WITH TESTICULAR TUMORS	NO. OF CRYPTORCHID PTS.	%
Gilbert and Hamilton (1940)	7,000	840	12.0
Campbell (1942)	1,422	165	11.6
Gordon-Taylor and Wyndham (1947)	636	82	12.9
Harnett (1952)	63	8	12.7
Schwartz and Reed (1956)	167	15	9.0
Thurzo and Pinter (1961)	142	9	6.3
Field (1962)	135	9	6.6
Hope-Stone et al. (1963)	282	17	6.0
Collins and Pugh (1964)	995	58	5.8
Dow and Mostofi (1967)	2,100	73	3.5
Johnson et al. (1968)	147	12	8.2
Total	13,089	1,288	9.8

°From Martin, D.C.: *J. Urol.* 121:422, 1979. © 1979, The Williams & Wilkins Co., Baltimore.

served incidence of 9.8% ($0.28 \times 35 = 9.8$). This view has been corroborated by several other authors, who showed the probability of a malignancy in an undescended testis as being 20 to 46 times greater than in a normally located scrotal testis.[9-13]

These figures represent a combined risk for all cryptorchid males, irrespective of the location of the gonad. Campbell[11] also found that although most undescended testes were located in the low inguinal region, the 14.5% of those located intra-abdominally constituted 48.5% of the testes in which malignancy occurred. Thus there is a six times greater risk for the testis situated in the intra-abdominal position to become malignant than for the lower-lying cryptorchid testis. It therefore appears that a direct correlation may exist between the degree of dysgenesis of the seminiferous tubules and the development of malignancy.[14] The higher incidence of dysgenic tissue in cryptorchid testes may account for the relative vulnerability to malignant degeneration.[15, 16] If dysgenesis is a factor in testicular tumorigenesis, dysgenic tissue in the contralateral scrotal testis might be associated with a higher incidence of malignancy than that in a normal scrotal testis. It is not surprising, therefore, that several authors have noted an increased incidence of neoplasia in the contralateral descended testis in patients with unilateral undescent.[5, 13, 17-19]

When patients with unilateral cryptorchidism had a germinal cell tumor, 95% of these tumors were reported to occur in the undescended testis.[10] An exception to this observation is the report by Gehring et al.[20]; they encountered seven tumors in the descended testis in 29 patients with a unilateral undescended testis who had a germinal cell tumor. Other authors noted that about one of five testicular tumors in patients with unilateral undescent developed in the contralateral scrotal testis.[1]

Bilateral undescended testes constitute about 10%[21] to 25%[22] of all cases of cryptorchidism. When patients with bilateral undescent have testicular tumors, 25% will have bilateral tumors.[11]

All of these observations contribute substantial evidence that undescended testes are at increased risk of malignant degeneration. The location of the testis appears to have a significant influence on this risk. The higher incidence of tumor in the undescended testis of the patient with unilateral undescent suggests that malignancy is related to the testicular position and not that the patient is generally cancer prone.

CAUSE OF MALIGNANCY

Although the correlation of germinal cell tumors with undescended testes has been amply documented, the etiologic mechanism remains unknown. The variation in chromosomal number and shape in malignant cells from different tissue organs has been well recognized. Mininberg and Bingol,[23] who reported that similar chromosomal abnormalities were present in the testicular biopsies of nine of 13 cryptorchid patients, suggested that these changes were related to failure of descent. On the other hand, Dewald et al.[24] from the Mayo Clinic were unable to find chromosomal abnormalities in any of the undescended testes among 13 boys studied. Indeed, their series provided no evidence to explain the propensity for subsequent malignant degeneration.

The failure of the germinal epithelium to mature and produce spermatozoa in locations other than the scrotum suggests that the location and environmental temperature may be significant factors influencing malignant degeneration. Dorman et al.[25] have reported the early findings of carcinoma in situ in the biopsy of an undescended testis in a 13-year-old child, implying that there may be a long latent period before the clinical manifestations of malignancy develop.

Several authors have reported the frequent occurrence of malignancy in atrophic testes regardless of the cause, suggesting that the hypoplastic nature of the cryptorchid gonad may be a causative factor in tumorigenesis.[26] Untreated undescended testes usually remain small and become hypoplastic or atrophic.

Testicular malignancy is a disease of young adults; the mean age of incidence is 32 years.[27] However, tumors occurring in undescended testes have a mean age of occurrence about 10 years later, suggesting that the etiologic factors may be different.

CARCINOMA IN SITU

Krabbe et al.[28] in Copenhagen performed testicular biopsies in 50 men previously treated for undescended testes, three of whom had a pattern of carcinoma in situ. Another man underwent orchiectomy for overt carcinoma. Patients in whom biopsy was done ranged in age from 18 to 35 years, but the age at orchiopexy for those with carcinoma in situ and the one with overt carcinoma ranged from 12 to 15 years. For the entire series, the age at detection of malignancy ranged from 13 to 26 years. A patient with carcinoma in situ reported by Dorman et al.[25] was 13 years old.

These reports suggest that malignant changes occur well in advance of overt tumors. Routine biopsy of all undescended testes may further elucidate this occurrence. It is possible that early treatment with orchiopexy by age two might alter the incidence of malignant change.

TORSION AND MALIGNANCY

Torsion is a well-recognized complication of the untreated undescended testis (see Chapter 10). In adults there is a high incidence of malignancy in testes that undergo torsion. Riegler[29] reviewed the literature and found torsion to be associated with malignancy in 64% of adult patients.

TUMOR CELL TYPE IN UNDESCENDED TESTES

The distribution of cell types among germinal cell tumors in undescended testes is somewhat different when compared with scrotal testes. Seminoma constitutes 30–40% of germinal tumors in scrotal testes but 60% in undescended testes.[6, 30] Teratocarcinomas, embryonal carcinomas, and occasional adult teratomas are other malignancies that have been reported most frequently with testicular undescent.

CLINICAL STAGE AND PROGNOSIS

A recent survey of 125 patients with tumors in undescended testes at Memorial Hospital in New York revealed that there were 42 patients in whom the testis was located in the scrotum at the time a tumor was found and 83 patients with uncorrected cryptorchidism.[31] At the time of diagnosis, 53% of these patients were in clinical stage I, 18% in clinical stage II, and 29% in clinical stage III. These findings are interesting, since some delay in diagnosis might be anticipated for testes not in the scrotum. The testis residing in the scrotum is favorably positioned for early recognition of anatomical change through ready access to palpation.

The five-year survival rate for all cell types and all clinical stages of testicular tumor was 62% in the Memorial Hospital series. This closely parallels the outcome from tumors occurring in descended testes; the review covered many years and encompassed an era when chemotherapy was less effective than it is now.

UNDESCENDED TESTES INITIALLY
SEEN AFTER PUBERTY

Patients with unilateral undescent that is first observed after puberty raise unique considerations in management. The adolescent cryptorchid testis is unlikely to mature for reproductive function even if orchiopexy is performed. Untreated, it provides endocrine function but exposes the patient to the risk of malignancy. If malignancy develops, the mortality may be calculated on the basis of the percentage of seminomatous and nonseminomatous tumors, due to the present excellent results of surgery, radiation, and chemotherapy. Martin and Menck[32] compared the risk of death with that of simple orchiectomy. The only available data for estimating the risk for orchiectomy came from the National Halothane study (National Science Foundation), which found the mortality associated with all anesthetics administered to patients undergoing such low-risk operations as herniorrhaphy, hysterectomy, and dental extractions to be 0.23% The risk of testicular malignancy varies with age and therefore these authors calculated the risk for various ages. Intra-abdominal and inguinal undescended testes were calculated separately because of the much higher malignant potential in the former. It was concluded that undescended testes recognized after puberty and before age 50 should be prophylactically removed, particularly if the gonad is atrophic and/or resides high in the inguinal canal or in the abdomen.[32]

Following the same reasoning, other authors have recommended orchiectomy for patients with unilateral cryptorchidism who have not undergone orchiopexy before puberty.[33] The risk of death due to malignancy is greater than that from surgical excision (Fig 13 – 1). When the testis cannot be identified at the time of inguinal exploration, in-

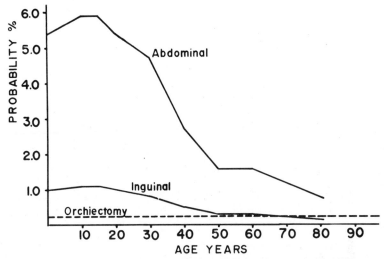

Fig 13–1.—Comparison of probability of death due to germinal cell carcinoma of testis in patients with abdominally and inguinally located undescended testes. The risk of death owing to orchiectomy is estimated from the National Halothane study of risk of anesthesia in "low-risk" operative procedures. (From Martin and Menck, *J. Urol.* 114:77, 1975. © 1975, Williams & Wilkins Co., Baltimore. Used with permission.)

traperitoneal exploration in this rare situation is particularly important to rule out the presence of a high abdominal testis. If an atrophic intra-abdominal testis is found, regardless of the patient's age it is wise to remove the gonad rather than attempt to place it in the scrotum, because the malignant potential is so great.

The patient who is first seen with bilateral undescended testes after puberty presents additional problems. Bilateral orchiectomy as cancer prophylaxis deprives the patient of almost all endogenous testosterone production, an undesirable state. Although there is no definite evidence that orchiopexy protects against malignant degeneration, a scrotal testis is more accessible for early detection of malignant growth. All high-residing testes identified at this late age are best removed, but the patient with bilateral low-lying testes might be advised to undergo orchiopexy of at least one testis for the purpose of better surveillance, followed by contralateral orchiectomy. Optimal management of this situation is highly controversial, and currently there is little solid evidence to support one approach over another. Indeed, some surgeons believe that no operative intervention is indicated under these circumstances. Bilateral orchiectomy produces the undesirable state of androgen deficiency, although hormonal replacement therapy is readily available and many prefer this to the risk of testicular malignancy.

ALTERED LYMPHATIC PATHWAYS

Lymphatic pathways from the testis may be altered in patients who have undergone orchiopexy or inguinal or scrotal surgery. The primary lymph nodes draining the testis may be located in the inguinal region rather than in the usual retroperitoneal area. Wittus et al.,[34] Herr et al.,[35] and others have described patients who had undergone prior orchiopexy in whom the inguinal lymph nodes were the primary site of metastases of testis tumors. Clearly, a therapeutic plan for the patient with a testicular tumor subsequent to surgery must include treatment of the ipsilateral inguinal nodes. In a patient with seminoma, the inguinal nodes should be included in the radiation field. The patient with a nonseminomatous tumor should undergo resection of the inguinal nodes, with standard retroperitoneal node dissection or at least a careful and frequent examination of the inguinal region after orchiectomy, since the inguinal nodes are relatively accessible for physical examination. We have resected both the inguinal and retroperitoneal nodes in most patients with germinal cell tumors of the testis who have undergone prior orchiopexy, even though in more than half of these patients the inguinal nodes were the only site of metastasis.

TUMORS AFTER ORCHIOPEXY

Frequent reports of testicular tumors occurring after orchiopexy have led most authors to conclude that placement of the gonad in the scrotum conveys no protection against subsequent malignant degeneration. Although this may be true, there is increasing evidence to challenge this long-held concept. The initial report of malignant testicular tumor is credited by some authors to Chevassu.[9] Our careful review of his original report revealed that after orchiopexy the tumor was present in the inguinal region, implying failure of the orchiopexy to secure the undescended testis permanently in the scrotum.[16]

In an extensive literature review on the subject published in 1978, my colleagues and I[9] identified 220 reported cases of germinal cell tumors that had occurred subsequent to orchiopexy. Among these reports were 97 cases described in sufficient detail to confirm that the orchiopexy had caused the testis to remain in the scrotum permanently. In other cases, the tumors were actually found in the abdomen, in

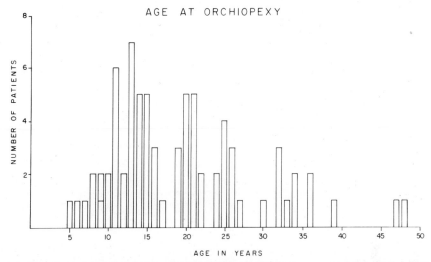

Fig 13–2.—Graph showing age at which orchiopexy was performed on 97 patients who subsequently had malignant tumor of the testis. (From Martin, *J. Urol.* 121:422, 1979. © 1979, Williams & Wilkins Co., Baltimore. Used with permission.)

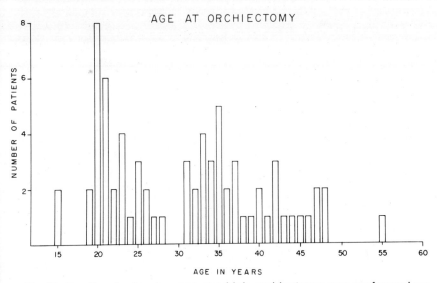

Fig 13–3.—Graph showing age at which orchiectomy was performed on 97 patients with well-documented germinal malignancies occurring after orchiopexy. (From Martin, *J. Urol.* 141:422, 1979. © 1979, Williams & Wilkins Co., Baltimore. Used with permission.)

the inguinal region, or in sites not specified. Because many tumors that appeared subsequent to orchiopexy were clearly not in testes secured in the scrotum, we accepted only 97 as properly documented cases. The age of the patients at the time of orchiopexy ranged from five to 48 years (Fig 13–2); it is significant that in only six of these 97 patients was the orchiopexy performed before age 10. Figure 13–3 shows the age at the time of orchiectomy for each of the 97 patients. The interval between orchiopexy and recognition of the malignant testicular tumor is diagrammed in Figure 13–4. It is noteworthy that in nine patients, this interval was less than 10 months; the mean period between orchiopexy and tumor diagnosis was 10 years.

It is very likely that many patients with undescended testes have undergone orchiopexy before age 10, and yet only six cases have been found in whom a subsequent germinal tumor developed. Although surgical repair of cryptorchidism before age 10 has become commonplace only during the past two decades, this observation suggests that early orchiopexy may be associated with a decreased risk of subsequent tumor formation. To confirm this hypothesis, we would have to

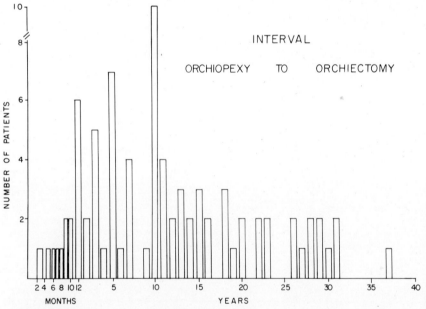

Fig 13–4.—Graph showing interval between orchiopexy and orchiectomy in patients with germinal tumors. (From Martin, *J. Urol.* 141:422, 1979. © 1979, Williams & Wilkins Co., Baltimore. Used with permission.)

TABLE 13-2.—TUMOR TYPES AFTER ORCHIOPEXY°

CELL TYPE	NO. OF TUMORS	%
Seminoma	34	40
Embryonal cell carcinoma	21	25
Teratoma	7	8
Teratocarcinoma	16	19
Embryonal cell carcinoma and teratocarcinoma	4	5
Embryonal cell carcinoma and choriocarcinoma	1	1
Teratocarcinoma and choriocarcinoma	1	1
Total	84	

°From Martin, D.C.: *J. Urol.* 121:422, 1979. © 1979, The Williams & Wilkins Co., Baltimore.

know the number of patients at risk. Currently we have no data to establish this information.

Is there an analogous observation in clinical medicine? There well may be. Carcinoma of the penis is extremely rare after circumcision in infancy, but the risk is not significantly reduced if circumcision is performed at puberty. A similar sequence may be postulated for the undescended testis. Early orchiopexy at one to two years of age, currently advocated by many surgeons, may allow full maturation of the testis and significantly reduce the risk of later tumor formation.

The incidence of cell type of tumors occurring after orchiopexy is comparable to that of cell types among normally descended testes. Seminoma does not predominate to the extent described for all undescended testes, as previously mentioned in this chapter. Table 13-2 shows the distribution of cell types in 84 reported tumors after orchiopexy.[9]

All patients and their parents should be advised that careful periodic examination of both scrotal compartments must be done throughout the patient's life, particularly during the third and fourth decades when tumors are most prevalent, whether or not an orchiopexy has been performed. Typical symptoms of testicular tumors in cryptorchid patients include pain and/or enlargement of the dystopic testis, abdominal or low back pain, abdominal mass, and leg swelling. It is difficult to determine from previous reports whether a direct relationship exists between infertility in cryptorchid males and subsequent development of testicular malignancy, although such a correlation is likely.[36]

Case Report

A 22-year-old man presented to University of California, Irvine, Medical Center with a six-month history of an enlarging right testicular mass. He had undergone bilateral orchiopexy at age 13. A radical orchiectomy now revealed embryonal cell carcinoma involving a large superficial inguinal node, and a bilateral retroperitoneal lymph node dissection disclosed multiple positive lymph nodes. Despite subsequent radical groin dissection and treatment with chemotherapy, the patient ultimately died of carcinoma.

This case illustrates several points discussed in this chapter. (1) Age 13 is far beyond the currently recommended time for treatment of undescended testes. We believe that early treatment will eliminate or reduce the occurrence of subsequent malignant change. (2) Biopsy of the testis during orchiopexy at age 13 might have revealed a carcinoma in situ pattern that would have directed the surgeon to orchiectomy rather than orchiopexy. (3) Presence of tumors after orchiopexy or other scrotal or inguinal surgery may alter the lymphatic pathways of the testis in such a way that the inguinal lymph nodes become the primary site of metastasis.

CONCLUSIONS

A comprehensive review of the literature on the subject of cryptorchidism and malignancy leads to several conclusions:

1. The cryptorchid testis is at increased risk of subsequent malignant degeneration.

2. Orchiectomy incurs less risk than a malignant tumor in patients with undescended testis who are first seen after puberty.

3. All patients with an undescended testis must be observed carefully for possible tumor, whether the testis is placed in the scrotum or not.

4. Early orchiopexy may provide some protection against subsequent malignant degeneration.

5. Tumors occurring after orchiopexy may spread initially to the inguinal lymph nodes.

6. Biopsy of the undescended testis is indicated for older patients in whom orchiopexy is planned.

REFERENCES

1. Johnson D.C., Woodhead D.M., Pohl D.R.: Cryptorchidism and testicular tumorigenesis. *Surgery* 63:919, 1968.
2. Carroll W.A.: Malignancy in cryptorchidism. *J. Urol.* 61:396, 1949.

REFERENCES

155

3. Rusche C.: Testicular tumors: Clinical data on 131 cases. *J. Urol.* 68:348, 1952.
4. Green R., Herr H., Scott M., et al.: Cryptorchidism and testicular neoplasia. *J. Natl. Med. Assoc.* 70:659, 1978.
5. Campbell H.E.: The incidence of malignant growth of the undescended testicle: A reply and re-evaluation. *J. Urol.* 81:663, 1959.
6. Collins D.H., Pugh R.C.B.: Classification and frequency of testicular tumors. *Br. J. Urol.* 36:1, 1964.
7. Grove J.S.: The cryptorchid problem. *J. Urol.* 71:735, 1954.
8. Whitaker R.H.: Management of the undescended testis. *Br. J. Hosp. Med.* 4:25, 1970.
9. Martin D.C.: Germinal cell tumors of the testis after orchiopexy. *J. Urol.* 121:422, 1979.
10. Gilbert J.B., Hamilton J.B.: Incidence and nature of tumors in ectopic testes. *Surg. Gynecol. Obstet.* 71:731, 1940.
11. Campbell H.E.: Incidence of malignant growth of the undescended testicle. *Arch. Surg.* 44:353, 1942.
12. Dow J.A., Mostofi F.K.: Testicular tumors following orchiopexy. *South. Med. J.* 60:193, 1967.
13. Thurzo R., Pinter J.: Cryptorchidism and malignancy in men and animals. *Urol. Int.* 11:216, 1961.
14. Sohval A.R.: Histopathology of cryptorchidism. *Am. J. Med.* 16:346, 1954.
15. Sohval A.R.: Testicular dysgenesis as an etiologic factor in cryptorchidism. *J. Urol.* 72:693, 1954.
16. Hope-Stone H.F., Blandy J.P., Dayan A.D.: Treatment of tumors of the testis. *Br. Med. J.* 5336:984, 1963.
17. Altman B.L., Malament M.: Carcinoma of the testis following orchiopexy. *J. Urol.* 97:498, 1967.
18. Field T.E.: Malignancy and the ectopic testicle in Army patients. *J.R. Army Med. Corps* 108:188, 1962.
19. Schwartz J.W., Reed J.F. Jr.: The pathology of cryptorchidism. *J. Urol.* 76:429, 1956.
20. Gehring G.G., Rodriguez F.R., Woodhead D.M.: Malignant degeneration of cryptorchid testes following orchiopexy. *J. Urol.* 112:354, 1974.
21. Snyder W.H. Jr., Chaffin L.: Surgical management of undescended testes. *J.A.M.A.* 157:129, 1955.
22. Gross R.E., Jewett T.C. Jr.: Surgical experiences from 1222 operations for undescended testes. *J.A.M.A.* 160:634, 1956.
23. Mininberg D.T., Bingol N.: Chromosomal abnormalities in undescended testes. *Urology* 1:98, 1973.
24. Dewald G.W., Kelalis P.P., Gordon H.: Chromosomal studies in cryptorchidism. *J. Urol.* 117:110, 1977.
25. Dorman S., Trainer T.D., Lefke D., et al.: Incipient germ cell tumor in a cryptorchid testis. *Cancer* 44:1357, 1979.
26. Hausfeld K.F., Schrandt D.: Malignancy of the testis following atrophy. *J.Urol.* 94:69, 1965.
27. Colby F.H.: *Essential Urology.* Baltimore, Williams & Wilkins Co., 1956.
28. Krabbe S., Shakkeback N.E., Berthelsen J.G., et al.: High incidence of undetected neoplasia in maldescended testes. *Lancet* 1(8124):999, 1979.

29. Riegler H.C.: Torsion of intra-abdominal testis. *Surg. Clin. North Am.* 52: 371, 1972.
30. Sohval A.R.: Testicular dysgenesis in relation to neoplasm of the testicle. *J. Urol.* 75:285, 1956.
31. Batata M.A., Whitmore W.F. Jr.: Cryptorchidism and testicular cancer. *J. Urol.* In press.
32. Martin D.C., Menck H.R.: The undescended testis: Management after puberty. *J. Urol.* 114:77, 1975.
33. Cunningham J.H.: New growths developing in undescended testicles. *J. Urol.* 5:471, 1921.
34. Wittus W.S., Sloss J.H., Valk W.L.: Inguinal node metastases from testicular tumors developing after orchidopexy. *J. Urol.* 81:669, 1959.
35. Herr H.W., Silber I., Martin D.C.: Management of the inguinal lymph nodes in patients with testicular tumors following orchiopexy, inguinal, or scrotal surgery. *J. Urol.* 110:223, 1973.
36. Fonkalsrud E.W.: The undescended testis. *Curr. Probl. Surg.* 15:1, 1978.

14 / Hormonal Therapy for Undescended Testes

W. MENGEL, M.D.
D. KNORR, M.D.
F.A. ZIMMERMANN, M.D.

A REPORT IN 1931 by Schapiro et al.[1] of their successful treatment of cryptorchid patients with gonadotropic hormones initiated this concept for use by others. Today the administration of HCG is recognized by many physicians as an equivalent of or at least adjunctive therapy to surgical treatment of cryptorchidism.

Recently a new type of hormonal therapy delivered via a nasal spray has been developed (see Chapter 9). Treatment with HCG or LH-RH provides the only successful method of nonoperative managment of cryptorchidism.

PATHOPHYSIOLOGY OF THE UNDESCENDED TESTIS

In 1970 Gier and Marion[2] described testicular descent in the following general manner: In the first phase the nephroblastoma and the gonadal primordium move downward as a result of stimuli from the developing metanephros and retrogressing mesonephros. The caudal mesonephric ligament develops into the gubernacular cord by the 55th day of gestation. This ligament later extends from the caudal pole of the testis to the fundus of the scrotum. There are extensions of the ligament to the perineum, to the inner thigh, and to the penis. The testis subsequently descends toward the internal inguinal ring, which it reaches by the 150th day of development. At this time, the course through the inguinal canal into the scrotum is prepared, and the processus vaginalis passes the internal inguinal ring and reaches the lowest point of the scrotum.

Testicular descent then commences. After the testis reaches the internal ring, the gubernacular cord, the posterior gonadal ligament, and the epididymis are propulsed downward into the inguinal canal.

These three structures grow until they are as large as the adjacent testis. Thus, the inguinal ring is enlarged sufficiently to permit testicular descent through the ring, which is supported by pressure from the abdominal organs and by traction from the gubernacular cord. The inguinal ring tightens after the testis descends, and pressure from the internal and external oblique muscles propels the testis toward the external inguinal ring. The gubernacular cord becomes shorter and thicker. Testicular descent usually is completed between the seventh month of gestation and the date of delivery.[3]

In mature newborn males with testicular undescent, the testes descend in two thirds of cases within the first three months. However, after the first year of life, spontaneous descent is rare.

Little is known about the hormonal mechanisms that regulate testicular descent. Either the hypophyseal LH of the fetus or placental HCG is believed to stimulate androgen production. The first elevated HCG-plasma level occurs between the 10th and 12th weeks of pregnancy, as measured by radioimmunoassay. The second high HCG level occurs during the last three months.[4] During the entire pregnancy, HCG passes through the placental barrier and enters the fetus.[5, 6]

Both the embryonic and fetal testes have a fully developed Leydig cell population. Male phenotype is determined by androgen production by the Leydig cells. It is believed that the first Leydig cells are stimulated by placental HCG.

Concentration of HCG in the fetus is about 3% of the maternal level, which is considerably higher than the HCG dosage used in hormonal treatment of cryptorchidism. The exact role of hypophyseal hormones from the fetus is still unknown but they appear to have an important effect on descent. Anencephalic infants are far more likely to have undescended testes than are healthy newborn infants. Shortly after birth the first population of Leydig cells completely vanishes.

TYPES OF UNDESCENDED TESTES

An accurate diagnosis of the type of cryptorchidism present is essential to initiate correct treatment, whether conservative or surgical. Because many reports in the literature recording good results from conservative therapy are based on varying definitions of the type of testicular maldescent present, it is necessary to establish exact nomenclature and accurate documentation of the clinical findings. We agree with Oberniedermayr and Maier,[7] Maier and Spann,[8] Hecker et al.,[9] Bierich,[10] and Knorr[11] in recommending the following nomenclature:

Cryptorchidism: This includes all forms of undescended testes.

Abdominal testis: The abdominal testis cannot be detected by palpation. Embryologically, the peritoneum fails to extend into the inguinal canal and thus the function of the gubernacular cord is ineffective. Gier and Marion[2] suggest that delayed closure of the umbilicus may influence the development of intra-abdominal testes, since intra-abdominal pressure to move the testis into the inguinal canal may be insufficient. A distinction must be made between an abdominal testis and anorchism or aplasia.

Anorchism: This condition is unilateral or bilateral absence of testes and must be differentiated from aplasia of the testes. In patients with male phenotype, a sufficient Leydig cell population must be present, since female characteristics will develop somatically, despite the male chromosome status, in the absence of androgen.

Inguinal testis: The testis can be palpated within the inguinal canal but cannot be transposed into the scrotum. The internal ring is wide, but the external ring is tight. According to Gier and Marion,[2] incomplete descent is caused by delayed or absent peritoneal projection of the peritoneum into the inguinal canal. The tissues of the lower inguinal canal are fused, and the processus vaginalis cannot reach the fundus of the scrotum, resulting in incomplete testicular descent.

Sliding testis: The testis descends past the external ring, but peritoneal adhesions of the spermatic cord, especially of the spermatic vessels, prevent complete descent. Clinically the testis is palpable at the external inguinal ring. The examiner is able to manipulate the testis into the upper scrotum, but it retracts immediately after it is released.

Retractile testis: This condition is caused by a hyperactive cremaster muscle; the testis usually is situated in the inguinal canal. When the muscle relaxes, the testis returns to the scrotum. The retractile testis is a physiologic variant of the descended testis and needs no treatment.

Ectopic testis: The testis is diverted from its normal path of descent after passing the external ring if the gubernacular cord is too weak or is missing. Most often the testis resides on top of the aponeurosis of the external abdominal muscle.

The indications for conservative or surgical treatment of cryptorchid testes therefore depend on the type of maldescent. Sliding and low inguinal testes have the greatest opportunity to descend normally with conservative treatment. We believe that initially the primary therapy for an abdominal testis also should be conservative. Administration of HCG leads to enlargement and better vascularization of the testis, to growth of the spermatic cord, and probably to enlargement of the inguinal canal. [10] All these changes may facilitate repair if an operation is required later.

No therapy is necessary for retractile testes. Primary surgical repair is indicated for all cases of ectopic testes and for inguinal testes with accompanying inguinal hernias. Surgical repair also is necessary if the testis is lodged in the inguinal canal after a hernia repair. Moreover, we recommend operation if there has been no descent after two courses of HCG therapy, or when puberty has already commenced and yet descent fails to start under the influence of endogenous hormone production.

THERAPEUTIC RECOMMENDATIONS

Intramuscular administration of HCG has been effective in causing descent in many children with undescent. Development of the fetus, which already has been exposed to a high prenatal HCG level, is stimulated by HCG treatment after birth. HCG exclusively possesses interstitial cell-stimulating hormone (ICSH) properties, and thus it stimulates only the Leydig cells, which produce testosterone. The germininal structures of the testes are not altered by HCG therapy. There is better vascularization of the testis, the spermatic cord is lengthened, and the inguinal canal is enlarged by HCG. [10]

Intramuscular injection of a single dose of 1,000 IU of HCG in a six-year-old boy induces a biologically active level for three or four days. The World Health Organization recommends the following dosage schedule:

1. Infants under one year of age receive 250 IU of HCG twice weekly during a period of five weeks.

2. Children up to five years receive 500 IU of HCG twice weekly during a five-week period; between the sixth year of life and puberty, 1,000 IU of HCG is given twice weekly during a period of five weeks; however, we recommend therapy before age four.

If descent occurs before the course of therapy is finished, it is necessary to complete treatment because there is a strong likelihood of retraction of the testis to its previous position.

Since HCG therapy stimulates the Leydig cells, the plasma testosterone level rises almost to normal adult values. Increased numbers of erections, hyperemia of the genital area, and a slight macrogenitosomia become side effects of treatment. When the course of therapy is completed, testosterone values decrease and after three weeks return to infantile levels. Permanent premature puberty is not induced.

Oral administration of hypophyseal gonadotropins is ineffective, and parenteral administration fails to help because the hormonal action is too brief. Animal gonadotropins are not used for human treatment since they rapidly produce antibodies.

Testosterone preparations are contraindicated inasmuch as strong virilization, premature epiphyseal closure, and suppression of gonadal development would result.

It is possible that treatment with postmenopausal gonadotropin (HMG), which has ICSH and FSH properties as well, may be effective, although the data are still speculative.

RESULTS

Follow-up evaluation must be done six months after completion of successful therapy with HCG, since there is a 10% incidence of retraction. Moreover, periodic follow up during several years is necessary. If retraction occurs shortly after the first course of HCG treatment is finished, a second course should be given.

Bilateral cryptorchidism with testes that are not palpable creates a special situation. Either bilateral abdominal testes or anorchism may be present, and these two conditions can be differentiated by an HCG test. If there is sufficient gonadal tissue, testosterone levels in the urine and in the plasma increase five to twenty-fold. If not, bilateral anorchism is likely to be present, and some surgeons believe that operative intervention is then unnecessary.

Such patients become hypergonadotropic by age 10 or 11, indicating that the pituitary gland is attempting to stimulate the absent or nonfunctioning testes. Early substitution therapy with testosterone is therefore mandatory. The age for commencing testosterone therapy depends on when gonadotropins can be detected in the plasma or urine, usually at age 11 or 12 years. During the beginning of therapy, oral treatment is sufficient. To complete full maturation, therapy must be continued during three years, with a depot testosterone preparation (250 mg every three to four weeks intramuscularly). Permanent testosterone replacement may be given in oral form. With this treatment regimen, the patient's primary and secondary sex characteristics will be completely normal and he will have potentia coeundi.[12] Implantation of a testicular prosthesis is advised for psychologic reasons in these patients.

INDICATIONS

Before starting a course of HCG therapy, an exact diagnosis must be made to avoid risks and useless treatment. Hormone therapy for an ectopic testis is just as inappropriate as surgical repair of a sliding testis. A follow-up study of 833 patients who had undergone operative repair for cryptorchid testes showed that the testes in 96.5% were located in the scrotum and in 1.5% outside the scrotum; in 2% there was testicular atrophy.

These results indicate that the operation, even in pediatric surgical departments, involves a risk of about 2%.

LATE RESULTS

There are two criteria for successful therapy: a good anatomical result and ultimate fertility. Using HCG, it is possible to produce adequate descent of inguinal or sliding testes in 50% of cases. The follow-up study of Richter et al.[12] compared the late results of fertility after HCG therapy alone with combined hormonal and surgical therapy. In 121 patients who underwent treatment for maldescended testes before puberty, a spermatogram showed that HCG therapy caused complete descent in 78 and was unsuccessful in the other 43; 39% of all patients had normal spermatograms and have been fertile. The fertility rate was 46% in the 78 patients who were treated with HCG only and 25% in those who underwent surgical therapy. The latter group had not responded to HCG therapy and therefore represented patients with more severe testicular abnormalities than the group that responded to HCG. Furthermore, the patients were not randomly placed in study groups to exclude patient bias, as recommended in Chapter 16.

CONCLUSION

These results show that conservative treatment with HCG has an established place in the management of undescended testes and may serve as an adjunct to surgical repair. Hormonal and/or surgical therapy should be provided before the third or fourth year of life to maximize the likelihood of subsequent fertility.

REFERENCES

1. Schapiro B.: Der Kryptorchismus chirurgisch oder Hormonell zu Behandeln? *Dtsch. Med. Wochenschr.* 38:38, 1931.
2. Gier H.T., Marion G.B.: Development of the mammalian testis, in Johnson A.D., Gomes W.R., Vandemark N.L. (eds.): *The Testis*, vol. 1. New York and London, Academic Press, 1970.
3. Scorer C.G.: The descent of the testis. *Arch. Dis. Child.* 39:605, 1964.
4. Varma K., Larraga L., Selenkow H.A.: Radioimmunoassay of serum human chorionic gonadotropin during normal pregnancy. *Obstet. Gynecol.* 37:10, 1971.

5. Geiger W., Kaiser R., Franchimont P.: Comparative radioimmunological determination of human chorionic gonadotropin, human placental lactogen, growth hormone, and thyrotrophin in foetal and maternal blood after delivery. *Acta Endocrinol. (Copenh.)* 68:169, 1971.

6. Stahl M., Girard J.: Die hormonale Behandlung des kindlichen Hodenhochstandes und die immunogenen Eigenschaften von humanem Choriongonadotropin. *Schweiz. Med. Wochenschr.* 102:202, 1972.

7. Oberniedermayr A., Maier W.A.: Die Descensusstörungen des Hodens und ihre Versorgung. *Z. Kinderchir.* 1:97, 1964.

8. Maier W., Spann W.: Die Bedeutung der rechtzeitigen Behandlung des Hodenhochstandes fur die Fertilität. *Dtsch. Med. Wochenschr.* 87:1697, 1962.

9. Hecker W.C., Hienz H., Daum R., et al.: Zum Kryptorchismus-Problem. Vergleichende morphologische und statistische Untersuchungen an beiden Hoden bei ein und beidseitiger Dystopie. *Dtsch. Med. Wochenschr.* 92:786, 1967.

10. Bierich J.R.: Moderne Gesichtspunkte zum Problem des Hodenhochstandes. *Internist* 8:42, 1967.

11. Knorr D.: Diagnose und Therapie der Descensusstörungen des Hodens. *Paediatr. Prax.* 9:299, 1970.

12. Richter W., Proescholdt M., Butenandt O., et al.: Die Fertilität nach HCH Behandlung des Maldescensus Testis. *Klin. Wochenschr.* 54:467, 1976.

15 / Role of Human Chorionic Gonadotropin in the Management of Undescended Testes

ERIC W. FONKALSRUD, M.D.
BARBARA M. LIPPE, M.D.

A TESTIS THAT FAILS to descend spontaneously, or that cannot be manipulated into a low scrotal position after the age of nine to 12 months, should be considered cryptorchid and, as such, requires treatment. There is considerable disagreement, however, regarding what constitutes optimal therapy and at what age it should be provided. Proponents of watchful waiting until puberty quote the studies of Johnson,[1] Baumrucker,[2] and Ward and Hunter,[3] which record spontaneous descent at puberty. This approach, although common in the past, is rarely followed today because of the strong histologic evidence indicating failure of potential maturation of the cryptorchid testis that fails to descend into the scrotum before three to four years of age.[4]

The possible benefits of exogenously administered HCG in effecting the descent of cryptorchid testes are still controversial in the American literature. Engle[5] in 1932 initiated the use of hormone therapy based on experiments with macaque monkeys in which an extract of human pregnancy urine caused testicular enlargement and descent into the scrotum. Although these studies were performed in preadolescent animals in which the testis normally rests in a suprascrotal position, they encouraged other investigators to determine if a similar descent in cryptorchid human patients could be achieved by exogenous administration of HCG. Among enthusiasts recommending the use of hormone treatment during the past 35 years, success has ranged from 15% to 66% in producing testicular descent.[6-11]

One of the most enthusiastic reports came from Ehrlich et al.,[12] who retrospectively analyzed children treated at Columbia University

Hospital in New York City. Treatment consisted of 10,000 units of HCG given in a short course of 3,300 units every other day in three injections, or in a long course of 20 injections of 500 units given three times weekly for six and one-half weeks. Testicular descent occurred in 23% of all patients treated (33% for bilateral, and 16% for unilateral cryptorchidism). The treatment appeared to be most successful in boys under age five years, in whom 55% of bilateral and 24% of unilateral cryptorchid testes were found to descend. However, this study, like most others on this subject, suffers because the exact location of each testis before and after treatment was not clearly identified, and the classification was done by many different examiners. Currently Ehrlich[13] is much less enthusiastic about the use of HCG in the management of unilateral undescent, since it is his impression that even the 16% or less success rate in this group after a series of multiple injections in young children may be less desirable than having the child undergo a formal orchiopexy. Many patients, in our experience, have refused a course of preoperative HCG because of the required series of painful injections, the potential risks of treatment, and the low likelihood of good response.

Gross and Replogle,[14] Rea,[15] and many others have called attention to the fact that most of the "successful" results following hormone administration have been achieved in boys who had retractile testes that subsequently would have descended spontaneously when endogenous gonadotropic hormones were produced in sufficient quantity. These authors point out that the true cryptorchid testis may be mechanically anchored in its downward pathway and that this obstacle cannot be overcome by exogenous use of hormones. Although there is no evidence that placing retractile testes in the scrotum before puberty in any way improves the permanent function or the morphological appearance of these normal gonads, a course of HCG may distinguish these testes and prevent unnecessary orchiopexy.

Thompson and Heckel[16] conclude that gonadotropins cause descent of only those testes that ultimately would have descended without treatment. They advocate hormone administration merely as a method of distinguishing testes that are destined to descend spontaneously from those that will require orchiopexy. They also point out that gonadotropin administration, even when it fails to cause descent because it does not lengthen the spermatic artery, enlarges the testis and rapidly increases vascular flow and vascular size and thus facilitates subsequent surgery. Additionally, Richter et al.[17] have found that 26 of 35 children with bilateral undescent who received a trial of HCG therapy in early childhood without orchiopexy had sperm counts above 10[6]/m after age 17. Lattimer et al.[18] believe that HCG may be helpful in enlarging the badly underdeveloped scrotum before orchiopexy.

Rivarola et al.[19] and others recommend a trial course of HCG for all patients with high nonpalpable testes in addition to careful monitoring of plasma testosterone levels. Patients with anorchism demonstrate no change in testosterone levels, whereas those with even hypoplastic testes show an elevation. Thus there is increasing evidence to support the trial use of HCG as a test rather than as a longer course of therapy, especially in older pubertal males. In pubescent males who have shown evidence of virilization, further exogenous HCG administration usually is not helpful. In addition, hormone therapy produces varying degrees of precocious sexual development in most patients, particularly when large doses are used. Premature epiphyseal maturation is another untoward effect that occasionally may be precipitated by long-term hormone stimulation. Injudicious hormone treatment also is attended by the risk of seminiferous tubule degeneration and even atrophy of the retained undescended testis, particularly if high doses are given.[6, 20, 21]

Many different dosage schedules have been suggested, from as low as 100 IU twice weekly for periods up to six months, to as high as that recommended by Lattimer[22] of 4,000 IU of HCG intramuscularly every other day for three doses. Most physicians would favor a schedule of about 1,000–2,000 IU every other day for a total of 10,000 IU. Flinn and King[23] suggested giving 100 IU per pound of body weight per week during a three-week period. Knorr[24] has recommended a trial course of HCG in almost all males with cryptorchidism based on the age of the patient: under the age one year, 10 doses of 250 IU twice weekly; from age one to two, 10 doses of 500 IU twice weekly; and over age two, 10 doses of 700–1,000 IU twice weekly (see Chapter 14).

The response to hormone therapy usually is prompt—within a matter of a few days after completion of therapy. Based on these observations, we currently use the schema outlined in Table 15–1 in management of patients with cryptorchidism. Of note is that the combination of elevated basal gonadotropins[25] and a failure of testosterone level to rise after HCG [26] are diagnostic of anorchism and considered sufficient to avoid abdominal exploratory laparotomy. A testosterone response to HCG in the presence of elevated gonadotropin levels has been reported in a case in which no intra-abdominal testes could be found, presumably reflecting the presence of microscopic Leydig cells along the course of the spermatic vessels.[27] However, our ability to diagnose

TABLE 15–1.—Use of HCG in Evaluation of Patients with Cryptorchidism

CLINICAL PRESENTATION	AGE (YR)	HORMONE TESTING	HCG PROTOCOL	RECOMMENDATION
Unilateral	3	None	1,000 IU 3×/wk (total of 10 injections)	Surgery in week following HCG if descent has not occurred
Bilateral (high scrotal or inguinal location)	3	None	Same	Same
Bilateral (no palpable gonadal tissue)	3	Basal testosterone; repeat testosterone 24 hr after last injection	Same	Surgery, if gonads are palpable but still ectopic. Exploratory laparotomy if plasma testosterone level rises after HCG. Suspect anorchism if testosterone does not rise; repeat testing as per suspected anorchism protocol
Suspected anorchism	11–12 (peripubertal)	Basal FSH, LH, and testosterone Repeat testosterone 24 hr after last injection	3,000 IU every other day × 3 doses	If basal FSH and LH are abnormally high and testosterone level does not rise, anorchism is likely and exploratory surgery may not be necessary. If testosterone rises independently of FSH and LH, exploration is indicated

this rare condition without surgery still may not be adequate, and exploration would still be recommended for this unique combination of circumstances.

SUMMARY

Although exogenously administered HCG may be helpful in causing descent in occasional patients with bilateral cryptorchidism and may be helpful in causing descent in gonads that do not have a mechanical factor causing limitation of descent, there is no clear evidence in the United States that it enables most of the usual inguinal or abdominal undescended testes with short spermatic arteries to descend and remain permanently in the scrotum. There also is no clear evidence that hormone therapy improves testicular structure or fertility in cryptorchid males beyond that which would have occurred spontaneously at puberty. Nonetheless, recent studies in which HCG has been given during the first four years of life suggest that subsequent function of the gonad may be better than if hormones were not used. There also is no indication that hormone therapy will in any way affect closure of the commonly accompanying hernia. Because of the occasional adverse effects attendant on injudicious administration of gonadotropins, this treatment should be used cautiously with a definite protocol in mind in appropriately selected patients.

Testosterone administration has been reported to induce descent of cryptorchid testes in about one fourth of the patients in whom it has been used.[28, 29] The results achieved with androgen therapy, however, have been much less convincing than those obtained after use of gonadotropin; moreover the reported clinical experience is sparse. The most encouraging results with hormone therapy have been associated with administration of LH-RH analogues (see Chapter 9).

REFERENCES

1. Johnson W.W.: Cryptorchidism. *J.A.M.A.* 113:25, 1939.
2. Baumrucker G. O.: Incidence of testicle pathology. *Bull. U.S. Army Med. Dept.* 5:312, 1946.
3. Ward B., Hunter W.M.: The absent testicle: A report on a survey carried out among schoolboys in Nottingham. *Br. Med. J.* 5179:1110, 1960.
4. Mengel W., Hienz H.A., Sippe W.G., et al.: Studies on cryptorchidism: A comparison of histological findings in the germinative epithelium before and after the second year of life. *J. Pediatr. Surg.* 9:445, 1974.
5. Engle E.T.: Experimentally induced descent of the testis in the macaque monkey by hormones from the anterior pituitary and pregnancy urine. *Endocrinology* 16:513, 1932.
6. Barcat J.: L'ectopie testiculaire; statistique clinique et opératoire des ser-

vices de chirurgie infantile des enfants—malades de 1940 à 1950. *Mem. Acad. Chir.* 83:909, 1957.

7. Bishop P.M.F.: Studies in clinical endocrinology: V. The management of the undescended testicle. *Guy's Hosp. Rep.* 94:12, 1945.
8. Brosius W.L.: Clinical observations on the effects of A.P.L. (Antuitrin-S) in the testicle. *Endocrinology* 19:69, 1935.
9. Lapin J.H., Klein W., Goldman A.: Cryptorchidism. *J. Pediatr.* 22:175, 1943.
10. Rea C.E.: Fertility in cryptorchids. *Minn. Med.* 34:216, 1951.
11. Deming C.L.: The evaluation of hormonal therapy in cryptorchidism. *J. Urol.* 68:354, 1952.
12. Ehrlich R.M., Dougherty L.J., Tomashefsky P., et al.: Effect of gonadotropin in cryptorchidism. *J. Urol.* 102:793, 1969.
13. Ehrlich R.M.: Personal communication.
14. Gross R.E., Replogle R.L.: Treatment of the undescended testis: Opinions gained from 1767 operations. *Postgrad. Med. J.* 34:266, 1963.
15. Rea C.E.: Further report on the treatment of the undescended testes by hormonal therapy at the University of Minnesota Hospitals: A discussion of spontaneous descent of the testis and an evaluation of endocrine therapy in cryptorchidism. *Surgery* 7:828, 1940.
16. Thompson W.O., Heckel N.J.: Undescended testes: Present status of glandular treatment. *J.A.M.A.* 112:397, 1939.
17. Richter W., Proschold M., Butenandt O., et al.: Die Fertilitat nach HCG Behandlung des Maldescensus Testis. *Klin. Wochenschr.* 54:467, 1976.
18. Lattimer J.K., Smith A.M., Dougherty L.J., et al.: The optimum time to operate for cryptorchidism. *Pediatrics* 53:96, 1974.
19. Rivarola M.A., Bergada C., Cullen M.: HCG stimulation test in pre-pubertal boys with cryptorchidism, in bilateral anorchia, and in male pseudohermaphroditism. *J. Clin. Endocrinol. Metab.* 31:526, 1970.
20. Charney C.W., Wolgin W.: *Cryptorchidism.* New York, Hoeber Medical Division, Harper & Row, 1957.
21. Myers R.P., Kelalis P.P.: Cryptorchidism reassessed: Is there an optimal time for surgical correction? *Mayo Clin. Proc.* 48:94, 1973.
22. Lattimer J.K.: Reports on current investigations. *News Bull. Am. Acad. Pediatr.* 1:16, 1971.
23. Flinn R.A., King L.R.: Experiences with the midline transabdominal approach in orchiopexy. *Surg. Gynecol. Obstet.* 131:285, 1971.
24. Knorr D.: Personal communication.
25. Lee P.A., Hoffman W.H., White J.J., et al.: Serum gonadotropins in cryptorchidism: An indicator of functional testes. *Am. J. Dis. Child.* 127:530, 1974.
26. Levine L.S., New M.I.: Preoperative detection of hidden testes. *Am. J. Dis. Child.* 121:176, 1971.
27. Kirschner M.A., Jacobs J.B., Fraley E.E.: Bilateral anorchia with persistent testosterone production. *N. Engl. J. Med.* 282:240, 1970.
28. Hamilton J.B., Hubert G.: Effect of synthetic male hormone substance on descent of testicles in human cryptorchidism. *Proc. Soc. Exp. Biol. Med.* 39:4, 1938.
29. Zelson C., Steinitz E.: Treatment of cryptorchidism with male sex hormone. *J. Pediatr.* 15:522, 1939.

16 / Timing of Repair for Undescended Testes

W. MENGEL, M.D.
F.A. ZIMMERMANN, M.D.
W.CH. HECKER, M.D.

UNDESCENDED TESTES, unilateral or bilateral, occur in about 0.7% of all boys aged one year or older.[1] The etiologic mechanism of this condition is complex and, despite extensive research, is still not fully understood. It is, therefore, not surprising that controversy exists concerning appropriate therapy, the aim of which is eventual fertility. After identifying the exact type of testicular maldescent, the appropriate treatment may be conservative or surgical.

Three types of cryptorchidism may be distinguished pathogenically:

1. Primary dysgenic: Genetic defects, e.g., Klinefelter's syndrome, Turner's syndrome, and the Moon-Bardet-Biedl syndrome, in all of which the gonads fail to respond to the hypophyseal stimulus;[2] also fetal damage leading to anorchism or atrophy of the testes.

2. Endocrinologic: Lack of maternal gonadotropins during the last two months of pregnancy when descent usually takes place,[2] an inborn disorder of synthesizing testosterone,[3] or a hypothalamo-hypophyseal disturbance with reduced secretion of gonadotropin.[4, 5]

3. Anatomical: Tight inguinal canal, short vas deferens or spermatic vessels, or malformation of gubernacular cord—possibly stemming from endocrinologic disturbances.

With respect to the ultimate goal of fertility, the complex of undescended testes must be divided into two categories:

1. Well-developed: Mechanical or hormonal factors prevent descent, and the malposition produces secondary damage to the parenchyma of the testis.

2. Primary dysgenic: Because the malposition is caused by an underlying disorder, normal function with fertility cannot be expected despite therapy.

The incidence of maldescent is related to the age of the patient; in premature infants it is between 20% and 33%,[6-9] whereas 1.8–4% of mature newborn infants have unilateral or bilateral maldescent. Subsequent descent within the first year of life, however, occurs in most infants with originally undescended testes.[7]

We believe that after the first year of life every undescended testis is pathologic. The incidence of undescent during the second year is 0.7–1%, and similar figures have been reported in adults (0.3–0.86%).[10-12] We are now aware that damaging influences causing morphological changes in the undescended testis begin during the first two years. Until a decade ago it was believed that the physiologic growth of the young boy's testis occurred in distinct phases, within which there were no important morphological developmental changes.[13-15] In 1954 Robinson and Engle[14] reported these phases of normal testicular growth: the first, between birth and the fifth year of life, is followed by a growing phase extending to the 10th year, after which there is a maturing phase; the entire developmental cycle is completed by age 16, when normal spermatogenesis occurs.

As recently as 1972, this generally accepted view was questioned by Staedtler and Hartmann,[16] who examined the testes of dead boys between the ages of one and 10 years, measuring the weight of the testes and diameter of the seminiferous tubules and counting the spermatogonia. They observed that the young child's gonads reveal a linear development pattern even before puberty. This view was supported by Knorr,[17] who observed a steady increase in testosterone production. A lengthy controversy has existed regarding the age at which damage to a dystopic testis begins. A number of reported pathologic observations may have been interpreted incorrectly, since many authors may have been unaware of the normal linear pattern of testicular development. For many years cryptorchidism in early childhood was not treated, and there was little investigation into early influences on testicular maturation.

Another controversy, still ongoing, concerns whether congenital or primary injury can be distinguished from secondary morphological changes resulting from malposition. As long ago as 1929, Cooper[18] noted morphological damage in undescended testes as early as the third year of life. Because this observation was unheeded, it failed to stimulate further research in this area for several decades. Hedinger[19] in 1971 repeated the suggestion that testicular damage may occur at an early stage in cryptorchidism. After noting that the undescended testis exhibits severe damage by the fifth year, manifested primarily by retarded maturation of seminiferous tubules, he questioned whether developmental retardation did not begin earlier.

Hedinger[19] believed that testicular function could not be evaluated objectively by examining Leydig cells, since they are not well developed in the early stages. Because the extent and degree of fibrosis vary greatly, as does the degree of maturation, Hedinger recommended the spermatogonia count as a more objective measurement for evaluating testicular function (Fig 16–1). By using the spermatogonia count as well as a qualitative examination of the ultrastructure of the interstitial tissue, we were able to show the following results in 578 malpositioned testes: in almost all cases the undescended testes showed no histomorphological changes during the first two years of life. The mean values of the spermatogonia counts were in the normal range but, after the second year, the spermatogonia counts decreased significantly. The courses of the counts were within the range of 10, which means that they remained low until puberty (the lower limit for normal values is 30).

In 1979 Hedinger[20] evaluated 619 testicular biopsies from 450 boys with unilateral and bilateral cryptorchidism between the ages of two months and 10 years and noted that the mean spermatogonia counts during the first year of life were equal to those found in normally descended testes. A difference in the spermatogonia counts between

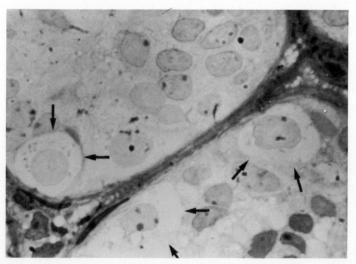

Fig 16–1.—Seminiferous tubules with spermatogonia *(arrows)*. Damage to testicular structures is demonstrable by counting spermatogonia in 50 cross sections of seminiferous tubules.[20]

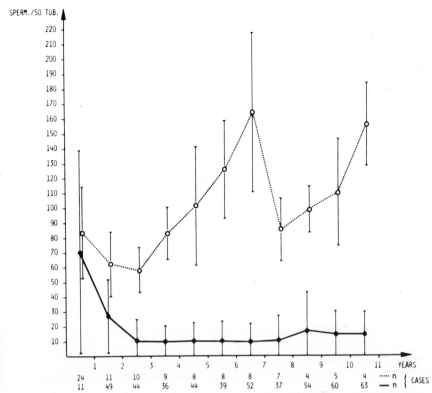

Fig 16−2. −Number of spermatogonia per 50 transverse sections of seminiferous tubules in all cryptorchid testes (•) and in normal controls (○): mean values per age group (for details see text). (From Hedinger, C.H.R., *Pediatr. Adolesc. Endocrinol.* 6:3, 1979. Used with permission.)

normal and cryptorchid testes was observed between the second and third years, but after the third year the mean spermatogonia values from cryptorchid testes were significantly lower than normal and remained at the same level until the beginning of puberty (Fig 16−2). There was no difference in spermatogonia counts between unilateral and bilateral cryptorchid testes of the same type. Both testes showed nearly identical mean spermatogonia values during the period of development (Fig 16−3). Hedinger[20] suggests that a reduced number of spermatogonia may be acquired during the early stages of development, although he never found complete absence of spermatogonia.

Electron microscopic examination of testicular connective tissue shows that with increasing age the undescended testis tends to degenerate, leading to enlargement and fibrosis. There is no difference in

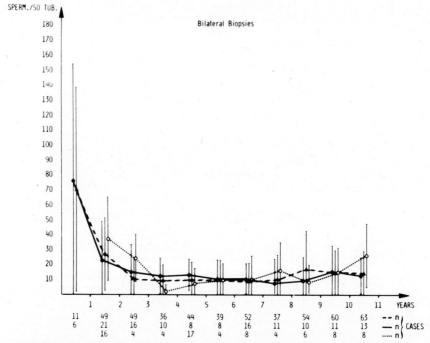

Fig 16–3.—Number of spermatogonia per 50 transverse sections of seminiferous tubules: mean values per age group in all cryptorchid testes (---) and in cryptorchid testes of bilateral (····) and unilateral (———) cryptorchidism. (From Hedinger, C.H.R., Pediatr. Adolesc. Endocrinol. 6:3, 1979. Used with permission.)

extent of interstitial tissue and in ultrastructural appearance between an undescended and a descended testis during the first year of life. However, after the fourth year marked fibrosis appears, with enlarged interstitial tissue of the undescended testis compared with that of bilateral descended testes (Figs 16–4 and 16–5).

Early ultrastructural pathomorphological changes in cryptorchid testes have been demonstrated in the second and third years of life.[21, 22] It remains unclear whether the underlying mechanism is a primary diminution of spermatogonia, with atrophy of the seminiferous tubules and secondary thickening and fibrosis, or an atrophy of the germinal epithelium due to diminished vascularization caused by the primary expansion of the connective tissue.

It has been of considerable clinical interest that not only the dystopic but also the contralateral descended testis shows pathomorpholog-

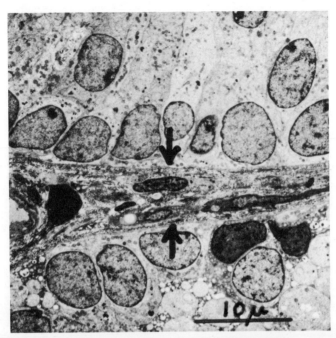

Fig 16—4.—Cryptorchid testis *(arrows)* of one-year-old boy. Thickness of interstitium is same as that of boy of same age with bilateral descended testes. Note scale with 10-μ measurement.

ical changes during the early years of childhood. The morphological changes in the orthotopic testis in patients with unilateral undescent have been reviewed by several authors, since biopsies have been routinely done on both the dystopic and orthotopic testes.

Zahor and Raboch,[23] Holzner and Gasser[24] and Bay et al.[25] found damage in the germinal epithelium of the orthotopic testis in 30–50% of cases of contralateral undescent. Hösli[26] showed such a marked decrease in spermatogonia counts in every sixth patient with unilateral undescent that subsequent infertility could be predicted. Using a morphometric test, Staedtler[27] showed that the spermatogonia count is lowered in both orthotopic and dystopic testes compared with controls.

Histologic examination of 262 biopsies from unilaterally descended testes in patients with contralateral undescent showed an abnormal germinal epithelium in 60.8% (Fig 16–6). We confirmed the observation by Hedinger[20] that the spermatogonia counts from unilaterally

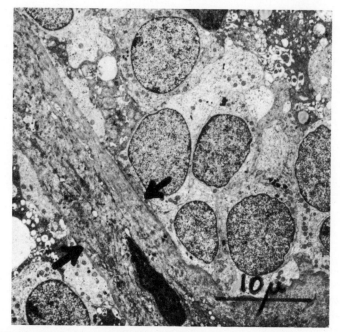

Fig 16–5.—Marked broadening of interstitium *(arrows)* in cryptorchid testis of four-year-old boy. Note 10-μ scale.

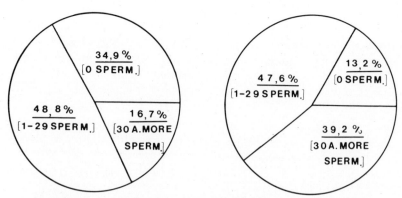

SPERMATOGONIA COUNT IN :

262 BIOPSIES
UNILATERALLY: DYSTOPIC

262 BIOPSIES
ORTHOTOPIC TESTES

34,9 %
[0 SPERM.]

48,8 %
[1-29 SPERM.]

16,7 %
[30 A.MORE SPERM.]

47,6 %
[1-29 SPERM.]

13,2 %
[0 SPERM.]

39,2 %
[30 A.MORE SPERM.]

Fig 16–6.—Spermatogonia count in unilateral cryptorchidism.

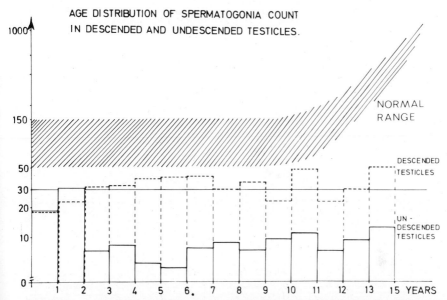

Fig 16–7.—Spermatogonia values in unilateral cryptorchidism during childhood.

descended testes are considerably higher than those from unilaterally undescended testes, but they have been lower than mean values from normal controls (Fig 16–7).

Experimental studies in mongrel dogs reported by Shirai et al.,[28] Weissbach and Ibach,[29] and Mengel[30] show that experimental malposition of one testis induces pathomorphological changes in the contralateral descended testis as measured by lower spermatogonia counts (Fig 16 –8,A).

Kiesewetter et al.,[31] Hecker,[32] and Kleinteich and Schickedanz[33] have demonstrated that children who undergo orchiopexy subsequently show an increase in the spermatogonia count. This clinical observation can be verified experimentally. In the dog with experimental unilateral cryptorchidism, a significant increase in the spermatogonia count can be demonstrated after scrotal orchiopexy (Fig 16–8,B).

The primary criterion for determining the success of treatment of cryptorchidism and the optimal date for initiating therapy is the late fertility, not merely the presence of a palpable testis in the scrotum.

It is difficult to compare the results among patients who have undergone different types of fertility studies following orchiopexy, but it is

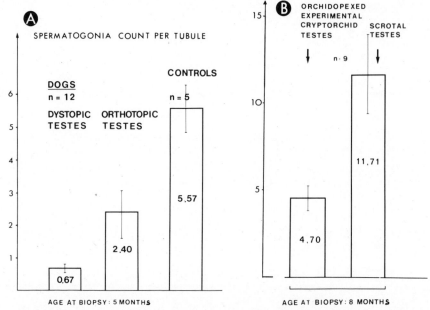

Fig 16–8.—A, spermatogonia count per tubule in experimental unilateral cryptorchidism of dog aged 5 months. **B,** same dog after orchiopexy three months later, showing maturation of germ cells in both testes.

apparent that the published fertility results are unsatisfactory (Tables 16–1 and 16–2).

In our patients, the operated on children had received HCG therapy beforehand and were therefore selected only if this therapy did not induce descent. The fertility rate reported by Knorr[1] after HCG therapy is 46% and is increased after orchiopexy by another 25%.

The main reason for the low fertility rates reported in the literature is that almost all of the patients did not receive treatment until after the age of six. We are now aware that such testes have already been extensively damaged during the first six years.

The follow-up study by Ludwig and Potempa[50] indicates the major role that proper timing plays in determining the success of treatment. In 71 patients who underwent orchiopexy for unilateral undescent between the first and the 13th years of life, the fertility rate correlates directly with an earlier date of operation. The fertility rate is 87.5% if orchiopexy is performed between the first and second years of life; it is lowered to 57% when the operation is performed between the third

TABLE 16-1.—Fertility in Bilateral Maldescended Testes

AUTHOR	NO. OF CASES	FERTILITY	SUBFERTILITY	INFERTILITY
Hansen (1946)[34]	25	8%	36%	56%
Alnor and				
Hartig (1954)[35]	11	9%		91%
Gross and				
Jewett (1956)[36]	16	75%	–	–
Hand (1956)[37]	49	63%	–	–
Nowakowski (1959)[38]	21	0%	19%	81%
Mack et al. (1961)[39]	27	7.4%	–	–
Maier and				
Spann (1962)[40]	25	20%	–	–
Knauth and				
Potempa (1963)[41]	6	0%	50%	50%
Bergstrand				
and Qvist (1964)[42]	35	35%	–	–
Eisenhut and				
Hohenfellner (1964)[43]	18	0%	22%	78%
Hortling et al. (1967)[44]	22	32%	55%	13%
Albescu et al. (1971)[45]				
Conservative	11	73%	–	27%
Operative	11	27%	–	73%
Pröscholdt (1972)[46]	49	27%	29%	42%
Kreibich and				
Köstler (1973)[47]	12	0%	50%	50%
Bramble et al. (1974)[48]	21	47.6%	–	–
Canlorbe (1974)[49]	7	14%	29%	57%
Ludwig and				
Potempa (1975)[50]	8	0%	–	100%

and fourth years, to 38.5% between the fifth and eighth years, and to as low as 25% between the ninth and 12th years. After the 13th year, the fertility rate is less than 14% (Fig 16-9).

SUMMARY

It is difficult in most patients to distinguish primarily damaged testes from those that are damaged secondarily. In the second and third years the first pathomorphological changes in testicular structures are apparent, as evidenced by reduction in spermatogonia count, retardation of tubular growth, thickening of interstitial tissues, and fibrosis.

The late fertility results after therapy for cryptorchidism reported in the literature are unsatisfactory. Most of these patients underwent orchiopexy after age six. The best late fertility results are obtained

TABLE 16-2.—FERTILITY IN UNILATERAL MALDESCENDED TESTES

AUTHOR	NO. OF CASES	FERTILITY	SUBFERTILITY	INFERTILITY
Hansen (1946)[34]	36	42%	50%	8%
Alnor and Hartig (1954)[35]	12	33%	–	67%
Hand (1956)[37]	101	46.5%		–
Knauth and Potempa (1963)[41]	12	33%	25%	42%
Doepfmer and Nienaber (1964)[11]	21	38%	43%	19%
Eisenhut and Hohenfellner (1964)[43]	15	0%	100%	0%
Hortling et al. (1967)[44]	19	74%	36%	0%
Albescu et al. (1971)[45]				
Conservative	7	100%	0%	0%
Operative	14	93%	–	7%
Madersbacher et al. (1972)[51]	36	25%	25%	50%
Pröscholdt (1972)[46]	72	46%	36%	18%
Kreibich and Köstler (1973)[47]	33	48%	52%	0%
Canlorbe (1974)[49]	8	38%	50%	12%
Ludwig and Potempa (1975)[50]	71	37%	0%	63%

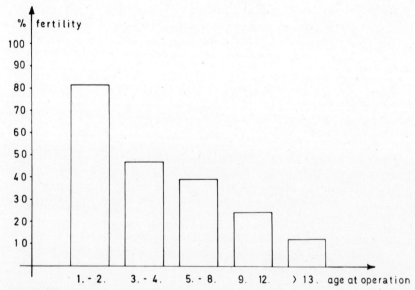

Fig 16–9.—Fertility in relation to age at operation in cryptorchidism. (From Ludwig and Potempa.[50])

when patients undergo treatment between the ages of one and two years.

Treatment of cryptorchidism before age one year is not necessary; operation is indicated only if there is concomitant incarcerated hernia or torsion of the testis. The second year is believed to be the best age to initiate treatment. Depending on the type of undescended testis, we recommend an initial course of HCG therapy and, for patients who do not respond, formal orchiopexy. Pathomorphological changes in the testicular structures produce abnormal spermatogenesis if treatment of cryptorchidism, whether unilateral or bilateral, is delayed beyond age five.

REFERENCES

1. Knorr D.: Fertility after HCG—treatment of maldescended testes in cryptorchidism: Diagnosis and treatment. *Pediatr. Adolesc. Endocrinol.* 6:215, 1979.
2. Bierich J.R.: Moderne Gesichtspunkte zum Problem des Hodenhochstandes. *Internist* 8:42, 1967.
3. Butenandt O., Knorr D.: Maldescensus Testis—konservative Behandlungsmöglichkeiten. *Dtsch. Ärzteblatt* 28:1799, 1977.
4. Job J.C., Garnier Ph.E., Chaussain J.L., et al.: Effect of synthetic luteinizing hormone-releasing hormone on the release of gonadotropins in hypophysogonadal disorders of children and adolescents. *J. Pediatr.* 84:371, 1974.
5. Prader A., Illig R., Zachmann M.: Prenatal LH-deficiency as possible cause of male pseudohermaphroditism, hypospadias, hypogenitalism and cryptorchidism. *Pediatr. Res.* 10:883, 1976.
6. Hofstatter R.: In Goerig K.H. (ed.): *Ergebnisse der Behandlung des Hodenhochstandes mit humanem Choriongonadotropin im Kindeshalter,* Inaug. dissertation, Munich, 1968.
7. Scorer C.G.: The descent of the testis. *Arch. Dis. Child.* 39:605, 1964.
8. Lange J.C.: Les cryptorchidies. *Ann. Pediatr.* 13:249, 1966.
9. Becker H., Gasteiger K.H.: Behandlung der Lageanomalien des Hodens. *Med. Klin.* 14:644, 1969.
10. Charney C.W.: The spermatogenic potential of the undescended testis before and after treatment. *J. Urol.* 83:697, 1960.
11. Doepfmer R., Nienaber W.: Die einseitige Hodendystopie (Kryptorchismus). *Münch. Med. Wochenschr.* 46:2096, 1964.
12. Frick J., Marberger H.: Zum problem der Retentio Testis. *Wien. Klin. Wochenschr.* 77:213, 1965.
13. Charney C.W., Conston A.S., Meranze D.R.: Development of the testis: A histological study from birth to maturity with some notes on abnormal variations. *Fertil. Steril.* 3:461, 1952.
14. Robinson J.N., Engle E.T.: Some observations on the cryptorchid testis. *J. Urol.* 71:726, 1954.
15. Mancini R.E., Rosemberg E., Cullen M., et al.: Cryptorchid and scrotal human testis: I. Cytological, cytochemical and quantitative studies. *J. Clin. Endocrinol.* 25:927, 1965.

16. Staedtler F., Hartmann R.: Histologische und morphometrische Untersuchungen zum präpuberalen Hodenwachstum bei normal entwickelten und zerebral Geschädigten knaben. *Dtsch. Med. Wochenschr.* 97:104, 1972.
17. Knorr D.: Uber die Ausscheidung vom freiem und Glucuron-Säuregebundenem Testosteron im Kindes und Reifungsalter. *Acta Endocrinol. (Copenh.)* 54:215, 1967.
18. Cooper E.R.A.: The histology of the retained testis in the human subject at different ages and its comparison with the scrotal testis. *J. Anat.* 64:5, 1929.
19. Hedinger C.H.R.: Uber den Zeitpunkt frühest erkennbarer Hodenveränderungen beim Kryptorchismus des Kleinkindes. *Verh. Dtsch. Ges. Pathol.* 55:172, 1971.
20. Hedinger C.H.R.: Histological data in cryptorchidism: cryptorchidism, diagnosis and treatment. *Pediatr. Adolesc. Endocrinol.* 6:3, 1979.
21. Hadžiselimović F.: Cryptorchidism: Ultrastructure of normal and cryptorchid testis development. *Adv. Anat. Embryol. Cell Biol.* 53(3):3, 1977.
22. Wronecki C.H.R.: In Slowikowski J., Zarzycki J., Sroeder J., et al.: Elektronenmikroskopische Untersuchungen am retinierten Hoden. *Z. Kinderchir.* 20:158, 1977.
23. Zahor Z., Raboch J.: Ein Beitrag zum Problem der Hodenbiopsie bei Kryptorchismus unter besonderer Berücksichtigung des Optimalalters für die Orchidopexie. *Schweiz. Med. Wochenschr.* 86:311, 1956.
24. Holzner H., Gasser G.: Hodenbiopsie bei Kryptorchismus. *Wien. Med. Wochenschr.* 116:311, 1966.
25. Bay V., Matthaes P., Schirren C.: Morphologische Befunde bei Hodenhochstand. *Chirurg* 39:331, 1968.
26. Hösli P.O.: Zur Problematik der Behandlung des Kryptorchismus. *Acta Urol.* 2:107, 1971.
27. Staedtler F.: *Die normale und gestörte präpuberale Hodenentwicklung des Menschen.* Stuttgart, Gustav Fischer-Verlag, 1973.
28. Shirai M., Matsushita S., Kagayama M., et al.: Histological changes of the scrotal testis in unilateral cryptorchidism. *Tohoku J. Exp. Med.* 90:363, 1966.
29. Weissbach L., Ibach B.: Neue Aspekte zur Bedeutung und Behandlung von Hodendescensusstörungen. *Klin. Paediatr.* 187(4):289, 1975.
30. Mengel W.: Klinische und experimentelle Studien zum Kryptorchismus-Problem. *Med. Habilitation, München,* 1978.
31. Kiesewetter W.B., Shull W.R., and Fettermann G.H.: Histological changes in the testis following anatomically successful orchidopexy. *J. Pediatr. Surg.* 4:59, 1969.
32. Hecker W.C.: Neue Gesichtspunkte zum Kryptorchismusproblem. *Münch. Med. Wochenschr.* 113:1125, 1971.
33. Kleinteich B., Schickedanz H.: Morphometric follow-up examinations of operated dystopic testicles. *Z. Kinderchir.* 20:261, 1977.
34. Hansen T.S.: Fertility in operatively treated and untreated cryptorchidism. *Acta Chir. Scand.* 94:117, 1946.
35. Alnor P., Hartig H.: Das funktionelle Ergebnis nach Kryptorchismusoperationen. *Chirurg* 25:294, 1954.

36. Gross R.E., Jewett T.C. Jr.: Surgical experiences from 1222 operations for undescended testis. *J.A.M.A.* 160:634, 1956.

37. Hand J.R.: Undescended testes: Report of 153 cases with evaluation of clinical findings, treatment, and results on follow-up to 33 years. *J. Urol.* 75:973, 1956.

38. Nowakowski H.: Der Hypogonadismus im Knaben und Mannesalter. *Inn. Med. N. F.* 12:1045, 1959.

39. Mack W.S., Scott L.S., Ferguson-Smith M.A., et al.: Ectopic testis and true undescended testis: A histological comparison. *J. Pathol.* 82:439, 1961.

40. Maier W., Spann W.: Die Bedeutung der rechtzeitigen Behandlung des Hodenhochstandes für die Fertilität. *Dtsch. Med. Wochenschr.* 87:1697, 1962.

41. Knauth H., Potempa J.: Hodenretention und Fertilität. *Urol. Int.* 15:77, 1963.

42. Bergstrand C.G., Qvist O.: Late prognosis in patients operated upon for bilateral cryptorchidism. *Symp. Int. Fertil. Assoc.* 25:4, 1964.

43. Eisenhut L., Hohenfellner R.: Die Spätergebnisse der Kryptorchis-musbehandlung und die resultierenden Folgerungen für die prophylaktische Medizin. *Ann. Paediatr.* 203:157, 1964.

44. Hortling H., de la Chapelle A., Johansson C.J., et al.: An endocrinologic follow-up study of operated cases of cryptorchidism. *J. Clin. Endocrinol. Metab.* 27:120, 1967.

45. Albescu J.Z., Bergada C., Cullen M.: Male fertility in patients treated for cryptorchidism before puberty. *Fertil. Steril.* 22:892, 1971.

46. Pröscholdt M.: *Spermatographische Nachuntersuchungen nach HCG-behandeltem Hodenhochstand.* Inaug. dissertation, Munich, 1972.

47. Kreibich H., Köstler H.: Der sogenannte Kryptorchismus aus chirurgischer und andrologischer Sicht. *Dtsch. Gesundheitsw* 28:67, 1973.

48. Bramble F.J., Houghton A.L., Eccles S., et al.: Reproductive and endocrine function after surgical treatment of bilateral cryptorchidism. *Lancet* 1:311, 1974.

49. Canlorbe P.: Problems of cryptorchidism. *Helv. Paediatr. Acta* [Suppl.] 34:47, 1974.

50. Ludwig G., Potempa J.: Der optimale Zeitpunkt der Behandlung des Kryptorchismus. *Dtsch. Med. Wochenschr.* 100:680, 1975.

51. Madersbacher H., Kövesdi S., Frick J.: Zur Fertilität beim einseitigen Kryptorchismus. *Urologe (A)* 11:210, 1972.

17 / Immunologic Aspects of Cryptorchidism

W. MENGEL, M.D.

F.A. ZIMMERMANN, M.D.

SEVERAL AUTHORS HAVE REPORTED large series of biopsies of undescended testes in which the cryptorchid testis was morphologically abnormal.[1-3] They described seminiferous tubules that developed pathomorphological changes leading to a disturbance in spermatogenesis with resultant infertility.

It has also been shown in biopsies of the contralateral descended testis in patients with unilateral undescent that pathologic changes are present in both testes and that they are similar.[3-9] Histologic studies performed on 262 biopsies of unilaterally descended testes from our clinic showed a normal epithelium in only 39.2% (Fig 17–1).

We employed an experimental model using eight-week-old mongrel dogs to determine the possibility of congenital damage in unilaterally undescended testes. During a period of three months, one testis in each of 12 dogs was surgically placed into the abdominal cavity, after which histologic examinations were carried out on both testes. The number of spermatogonia and the mean diameter of the seminiferous tubules were measured. These studies found that both testes showed a statistically significant decrease in each of these measurements compared with control dogs with bilaterally descended testes. The number of spermatogonia showed a deficit of 88% (0.67 spermatogonia per tubule; S/T) in the dystopic testis, and 56.9% (2.40 S/T) in the unilateral descended testis (Fig 17–2). The normal value is 5.57 S/T. Our results in clinical studies on unilaterally cryptorchid boys are similar to those of Shirai et al.[10] and Weissbach et al.[11, 12] The results from these studies strongly suggest that the etiologic mechanism of the abnormal testicular structure in cryptorchidism is not due primarily to congenital damage. The clinical fertility studies by Pröscholdt and Knorr[13] and Ludwig and Potempa[14] substantiate this view.

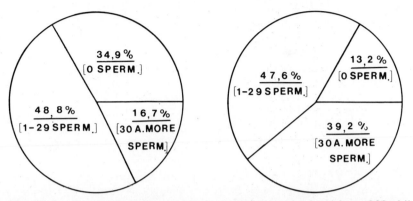

Fig 17–1.—Spermatogonia counts from biopsies obtained from 262 children with unilaterally undescended testes (50 tubules counted per biopsy). On left, unilateral dystopic testes; on right, orthotopic testes.

The question then arises as to how the damage in cryptorchid testes occurs, and whether the damage in the descended testis in patients with unilateral undescent could be caused by the abnormal undescended testis. There are many similarities between cases of clinical or experimental unilateral cryptorchidism and those of experimental al-

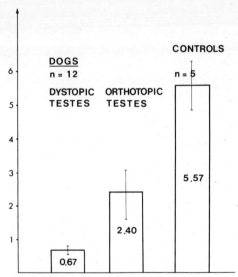

Fig 17–2.—Spermatogonia count in experimental unilateral cryptorchidism in dystopic and orthotopic descended testes.

lergic orchitis (EAO). Therefore, it is possible that a similar autosensitization against testicular tissue may be the reason for the damage in the unilateral cryptorchid and contralateral orthotopic testes.

IMMUNOLOGIC FEATURES OF THE TESTIS

The presence of spermatozoan autoantibodies has been recognized for a long time and has been shown in large series of patients with various testicular disorders.[15-22] On the other hand, autosensitization against other testicular structures has been demonstrated in only a few cases.

Isidori et al.[23, 24] and Dondero and Isidori[25] found antibodies against spermatozoa, germinal epithelium, tubular wall, and connective tissue in 12 of 48 patients with hypogonadism and infertility but without genetic disorders. Wall et al.[26] demonstrated antibodies against Sertoli cells in a patient with hypogonadism and azospermia; the striking histologic feature of this testis was a cessation of maturation. In a collective study of 93 fertile men, the same authors identified autoantibodies against germinal cells in 11% and against sperm in 26%. The histologic features of the testes in these patients were normal but showed a cessation of maturation. Finally, Murthy et al.[27] were able to demonstrate circulating antibodies against the basement membrane of the tubular wall, as well as against the germinal cells, in a patient with multiple endocrinologic disorders. The histologic picture from this testis showed a reduction of the germinal epithelium, fibrosis of the connective tissue, and destruction of the seminiferous tubules. It is interesting to note that Haensch[28] found a close correlation between the presence of autoantibodies against spermatozoa and conditions causing testicular dystopia. He identified dystopia of the testes in 50% of 858 patients with fertility problems.

Schoysmann[29] performed a unilateral orchiectomy on each of four patients with high spermagglutinin titers and accompanying unilateral testicular dystopia. At follow-up examination three years later, he found a marked decrease in spermagglutinin titers and normalization of the spermiogram in all patients.

According to the results of Johnson[30] and Tung et al.,[31, 32] the basement membrane of the seminiferous tubules acts as an immunologic barrier, which under normal circumstances prevents the penetration of antibodies into the seminiferous tubules. Under pathologic conditions, the basement membrane may become porous, and several parts of the seminiferous tubules may be exposed to antibodies, possibly leading to an antigen-antibody reaction.

EXPERIMENTAL ALLERGIC ORCHITIS

Since testicular maldescent and EAO have many manifestations in common, a discussion of the pathogenesis of EAO is of interest. In both conditions external influences damage the germinal epithelium and lead to suppression of spermatogenesis.

Voisin et al.[33] as well as Freund et al.[34] were able to create experimentally an allergic orchitis in guinea pigs, with resultant morphological changes in the seminiferous tubules. They injected homogenized testes emulsified in Freund's adjuvant, and only eight or nine days after immunization, morphological changes were demonstrable.

The following observations have been made in testes with EAO:

1. The spermatids are desquamated and their acrosomes are deformed, as seen in electron microscopy.[35, 36] Consequently, the later forms of spermatogenesis, except for the spermatogonia, disappear.

2. Seminiferous tubules and the rete testis are surrounded by lymphocytes and monocytes, which are attached to the basement membrane. Macrophages and lymphocytes penetrate the basement membrane and reach the lumen of the tubules as well as the Sertoli cells. In the early stages, the germinal cells and the Sertoli cells are unaffected by the macrophages, but later the complete cell population becomes desquamated, resulting in aspermatogenesis. The total inflammation presents a picture of monocytes, lymphocytes, eosinophilic cells, and polymorphonuclear cells, which are located on the vessels around the seminiferous tubules. Later there are only macrophages in the tubules.

3. In the draining ductules, in the head and tail of the epididymis, and in the vas deferens, polymorphonuclear cells are present.

Many authors stress that the aspermatogenesis associated with EAO may result from migration of humoral antibodies into the seminiferous tubules.[34, 37-40] Brown and Glynn[40] observed IgG in the acrosomes of the sperm as early as the fifth day after immunization, but Tung et al.[41] and Johnson[42] were unable to show this phenomenon.

Bishop[43] found, after sensitization of newborn guinea pigs with homogenized homologous testes and complete Freund's adjuvant, an early rise of antibodies and degenerative tubular changes, but aspermatogenesis was detected only after puberty. Inflammation was not observed.

Waksman,[44] Tung et al.,[41] and Johnson[30] suggested that the damage to the testis in EAO with infiltration of mononuclear cells is caused by a cell-mediated immunity. Johnson[42] found only traces of IgG next to the infiltrated mononuclear cells and could not detect antibodies against sperm in the region of the seminiferous ductules. On the other hand, Tung et al.[41] and Nagano and Okomura[36] were able to show binding of immunoglobulins and complement in the rete testis and in the tail of the epididymis.

From an immunologic point of view, there are different opinions regarding the causes of testicular damage in experimental EAO. Tung et al.[41] demonstrated in follow-up studies that the cellular infiltration does not begin before the ninth day after immunization. On the other hand, Nagano and Okomura[36] found that aspermatogenesis may occur in an early phase of EAO. Both reports demonstrated electron microscopic changes in testicular structure before the appearance of mononuclear infiltration.

Brown and Glynn[40] and Johnson[45] pointed out that the first change in EAO is the gathering of polymorphonuclear cells in the deferent ductules. They believe that, owing to this damage, the blood-testis barrier will be altered and humoral antibodies will enter the seminiferous tubules, resulting in aspermatogenesis. Waksman,[44] Tung et al.,[41] and Johnson[45] suggested that the damage from EAO is caused by a cellular immunoreaction in the seminiferous tubules and the rete testis. This reaction is characterized by a mononuclear infiltration, which leads eventually to aspermatogenesis. The varying results observed by several authors may be owing to the different animal species employed.[22]

In summarizing the literature, it becomes apparent that the blood-testis barrier (Johnson[45]) is the main factor in the origin of intratubular damage. The basis for the development of EAO appears to be the combination of testicular antigen and sensitized lymphocytes.

Tung and Alexander[46] discuss three possibilities regarding the cause of EAO:

1. Antibodies or lymphocytes enter the rete testis and have contact with antigens from sperm, which may cause an initial lesion. From there an ascending inflammation reaches the seminiferous tubules. The studies of Waksman[44] and Johnson[45] show that the earliest and most prominent lesions are present in the rete testis.

2. An unknown helper factor makes the blood-testis barrier permeable to immunoglobulins and T lymphocytes. The studies of Pokorna,[47] Voisin and Toullet,[48] and Willson et al.[49] show that complete Freund's adjuvant makes the blood-testis barrier permeable. They injected horseradish-peroxidase intravenously and were able to demonstrate its presence in the cytoplasm of spermatogonia and in Sertoli cells. It did not change the connection between the Sertoli cells.

3. The antibodies react with aspermatogenic antigens beyond the blood-testis barrier.

In summarizing the results from different studies, it may be stated that EAO is an organ-specific immunologic disease that leads to damage to spermatogenesis in both testes. The pathogenesis is characterized by a complex immunologic process that is dependent on whether the antibody or the sensitized lymphocyte makes contact with testicular antigen. It is very likely that humoral as well as cell-mediated immunologic reactions play a role and lead to the typical cellular lesions in testicular tissue (Tung[22]).

According to Johnson,[45] the blood-testis barrier seems to be the most important physiologic barrier and prevents permeation of immunocompetent cells into the intratubular structures.

This barrier exists between the vessels and the seminiferous tubules in the peritubular connective tissue. Tung[22] believes that the mechanism of intratubular damage in EAO is due to an unknown helper factor that destroys the blood-testis barrier. Thus lymphocytes may obtain direct contact with antigenic material in the seminiferous tubules. This mechanism can be discussed as a possible model for the unilateral cryptorchid testis with some assumptions.

It is widely reported that the environmental temperature in the abdominal cavity or the inguinal canal is 1–2 C higher than in the scrotum. The higher temperature is commonly regarded as the reason for the damage to an undescended testis. This widely accepted hypothesis has not been completely proved. Rapaport et al.[50] and Fernandez-Collazo et al.[51] were able to demonstrate in a guinea pig model that brief thermic alterations lead to marked morphological changes in both of the testes and to autoimmunoreactions as well. These changes are similar to those created in the model of EAO. The question arises whether a permanent unphysiologic temperature can achieve the same result as a short-term high temperature. According to the view of Tung,[22] it is possible that a permanent high unphysiologic environmental temperature makes the blood-testis barrier permeable for immune-competent cells. A helper factor may assist. This process may then produce an autoantibody reaction against testicular structures.

The hypothesis of an immunopathogenic origin of pathologic changes in cryptorchid testes is supported by our own experimental studies. Using the previously described model of experimental unilateral testicular maldescent in young mongrel dogs, we injected azathioprine as an immunosuppressive agent in a dosage of less than 7

TABLE 17–1.—INCREASE IN NUMBER OF SPERMATOGONIA IN
EXPERIMENTAL UNILATERAL CRYPTORCHIDISM WITH AZATHIOPRINE

POSITION OF TESTES	MEAN SPERMATOGONIA COUNT		INCREASE IN SPERMATOGONIA COUNT	SIGNIFICANCE
	DOGS WITH AZATHIOPRINE	DOGS WITHOUT AZATHIOPRINE		
Unilateral dystopic	1.48	0.67	120.9%	p = 0.01
Unilateral orthotopic	4.25	2.40	77.1%	p = 0.01

mg/kg of body weight. Azathioprine prevents both cellular and humoral immune reactions. This dosage does not interfere with the development of intratubular tissue (Seidenkranz et al.[52]). We found a statistically significant increase in spermatogonia in both the unilateral cryptorchid and the contralateral descended testis. With azathioprine treatment, the increase in the spermatogonia count is 120.9% for dystopic testes and 77.1% for orthotopic testes (Table 17–1) (Fig 17–3). The spermatogonia count of 4.25 in the orthotopic testes is not far from the normal spermatogonia value of 5.75.

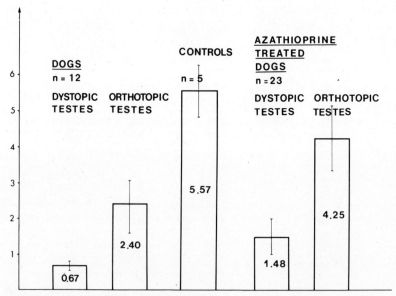

Fig 17–3.—Increase in spermatogonia count with azathioprine treatment in canine model of unilateral cryptorchidism.

SUMMARY

There are strong parallels between experimentally produced unilateral cryptorchidism in the dog model and the condition of patients with unilateral testicular maldescent. In both situations similar pathomorphological changes appear in both testes that can be verified by measuring the mean diameter of the tubules and the number of spermatogonia present.

The experimental studies described and the long-term results of early treatment of cryptorchidism exclude the possibility of a congenital defect as the cause of the dystopic changes in undescended testes. It is probable that the dystopic gonad is responsible for an induced disturbance that produces pathomorphological changes in both the undescended and orthotopic testis. These changes are due to autoimmune reactions against testicular tissue.

Application of azathioprine, which suppresses the cellular and humoral immune reactions, increases the number of spermatogonia of the dystopic and the orthotopic testes in our model of experimental unilateral cryptorchidism in dogs within three months. We stress that the mechanism of this hypothetical autoimmune reaction can be stopped by application of a potent immunosuppressive agent.

There are some parallels among experimental unilateral cryptorchidism, EAO, and the clinical features of unilateral testicular undescent:

1. In EAO, inflammation can be observed after immunization with homogenized testicular tissue in combination with the complete adjuvant of Freund and associates.[34] This inflammation tends to damage the intratubular structures.

2. In our canine model of unilateral cryptorchidism, we observed pathomorphological changes in both testes, retardation of tubular development, and disturbances of spermatogonia production.

Both conditions produce a similar form of damage to the germinal epithelium.

The cause of testicular damage in cryptorchidism is the higher environmental temperature in the abdomen or in the inguinal canal. As shown in the experiments of Rapaport et al.[50] and Fernandez-Collazo et al.,[51] high temperature can induce autoimmune reactions in the experimental model which may be the pathophysiologic mechanism of testicular damage.

The permanent unphysiologic elevation in testicular temperature makes the blood-testis barrier[45] of the cryptorchid testis permeable for immune-competent cells. A helper factor, as suggested by Tung[22] for the EAO model, may assist in this event. The result is an autoimmune reaction, with formation of autoantibodies against tubular tissue. The reaction takes place in both the orthotopic and dystopic testis, producing the extensive pathologic changes.

It is not clear why there are no cellular infiltrations in either the cryptorchid or the orthotopic testis three months after the start of the experiment. Cellular infiltrations are described for EAO by various authors.[33, 34, 38, 41, 44, 45] Cell infiltration may no longer be present after three months or the mechanism may be only humoral, as suggested by Tung.[22]

REFERENCES

1. Hedinger C.H.R.: Uber den Zeitpunkt frühest erkennbarer Hodenveränderungen beim Kryptorchismus des Kleinkindes. *Verh. Dtsch. Ges. Pathol.* 55:172, 1971.
2. Hecker W.C.: Neue Gesichtspunkte zum Kryptorchismus Problem. *Münch. Med. Wochenschr.* 113:1125, 1971.
3. Hösli P.O.: Zur Problematik der Behandlung des Kryptorchismus. *Acta Urol.* 2:107, 1971.
4. Raboch J., Zahor Z.: Ein Beitrag zum Studium der inkretonschen Hodenfunktion bei Kryptorchismus. *Endokrinologie* 33:160, 1956.
5. Nelson W.O.: Some problems of testicular function. *J. Urol.* 69:325, 1953.
6. Bay V., Matthaes P., Schirren C.: Morphologische Befunde bei Hodenhochstand. *Chirurg* 39:331, 1968.
7. Scott L.S.: Unilateral cryptorchidism: Subsequent effects on fertility. *J. Reprod. Fertil.* 2:54, 1961.
8. Holzner H., Gasser G.: Hodenbiopsie bei Kryptorchismus. *Wien Med. Wochenschr.* 116:311, 1966.
9. Städtler F.: Die normale und gestörte praepuberale Hodenentwicklung des Menschen. *Veroeff. Morphol. Pathol.* 92:1, 1973.
10. Shirai M., Matsushita S., Kagayama M., et al.: Histological changes of the scrotal testis in unilateral cryptorchidism. *Tohoku J. Exp. Med.* 90:363, 1966.
11. Weissbach L., Ibach B.: Neue Aspekte zur Bedeutung und Behandlung von Hodendescensusstörungen. *Klin. Paediatr.* 187:289, 1975.
12. Weissbach L., Müller R.: Histometrische Untersuchungen am puberalen Hundehoden beim experimentellen unilateralen Kryptorchismus. *Z. Kinderchir.* 16:53, 1975.
13. Pröscholdt M.: *Spermatographische Nachuntersuchungen nach HCG-behandeltem Hodenhochstand.* Inaug. dissertation, Munich, 1972.
14. Ludwig G., Potempa J.: Der optimale Zeitpunkt der Behandlung des Kryptorchismus. *Dtsch. Med. Wochenschr.* 100:680, 1975.
15. Hekman A., Rümke Ph.: The antigens of human seminal plasma: With special reference to lactoferrin as a spermatozoa-coating antigen. *Fertil. Steril.* 20:312, 1969.
16. Günther E.: Die immunologisch Bedingte Orchitis. *Andrologie* 4:157, 1972.

17. Shulman S., Zappi E., Ahmed U., et al.: Immunologic consequences of vasectomy. *Contraception* 5:269, 1972.
18. Ansbacher R.: Vasectomy: Sperm antibodies. *Fertil. Steril.* 24:788, 1973.
19. Haensch R.: Histologische Veränderungen der Lymphknoten nach endolymphatischer, Radiogold-Therapie. *Arch. Dermatol. Forsch.* 244:256, 1972.
20. Voisin G. A., Toullet F., D'Almeida M.: *Characterization of spermatozoal auto-, iso- and allo-antigens,* Karolinska symposia on research methods in reproductive endocrinology, 7. Stockholm, Symposium, July 1974, p. 173.
21. Friberg J., Kjessler B.: Sperm-agglutinating antibodies and testicular morphology in 59 men with azoospermia or cryptazoospermia. *Am. J. Obstet. Gynecol.* 121:987, 1975.
22. Tung K.S.K.: Human sperm antigens and antisperm antibodies: I. Studies on vasectomy patients. *Clin. Exp. Immunol.* 20:93, 1975.
23. Isidori A., Dondero F., Garufi L.A.: Rilieri di immunopatologica nel testicole umane. *Folia Endocrinol.* 21:271, 1968.
24. Isidori A., Dondero F., Lombardo D.: *Autoimmunization in male infertility,* Communication to 2d Int. Symp. on Immunology of Reproduction, Varna, 1971.
25. Dondero F., Isidori A.: Autoimmunisation antitesticulaire chez l'homme. *Ann. Endocrinol. (Paris)* 33:417, 1972.
26. Wall J.R., Stedronska J., Lessof M.H.: Antibodies against Sertoli cells in human infertility. *Clin. Endocrinol.* 3:187, 1974.
27. Murthy G.G., Peress N.S., Khan S.A.: Demonstration of antibodies to testicular basement membrane by immunofluorescence in a patient with multiple primary endocrine deficiencies. *J. Clin. Endocrinol. Metabol.* 42:637, 1976.
28. Haensch R.: Autoimmunpathologische Fertilitatsstorungen des Mannes. *Arch. Klin. Exp. Dermatol.* 237:61, 1970.
29. Schoysmann R.: The secondary male sterility. *Andrologie* 2:71, 1970.
30. Johnson M.H.: An immunological barrier in the guinea pig testis. *J. Pathol.* 101:129, 1970.
31. Tung K.S.K., Unanue E.R., Dixon F.J.: Pathogenesis of experimental allergic orchitis: I. Transfer with immune lymph node cells. *J. Immunol.* 106:1453, 1971.
32. Tung K.S.K., Unanue E.R., Dixon F.J.: Pathogenesis of experimental allergic orchitis: II. The role of antibody. *J. Immunol.* 106:1463, 1971.
33. Voisin G., Delaunay A., Barber M.: Sur des lesions testiculaires provoquées chez le cobaye par iso- et autosensibilization. *Ann. Inst. Pasteur* 81: 48, 1951.
34. Freund J., Lipton M.M., Thompson G.E.: Aspermatogenesis in the guinea pig induced by testicular tissue and adjuvants. *J. Exp. Med.* 97:711, 1953.
35. Brown P.C., Dorling J., Glynn L.E.: Ultrastructural changes in experimental allergic orchitis in guinea pigs. *J. Pathol.* 106:229, 1972.
36. Nagano T., Okomura K.: Fine structural changes of allergic aspermatogenesis in the guinea pig: I. The similarity in the initial changes induced by passive transfer of anti-testis serum and by immunization with testicular tissue. *Virchows Arch. [Pathol. Anat.]* 14:223, 1973.
37. Katsh S., Bishop D.W.: The effect of homologous testicular and brain and

heterologous testicular homogenates combined with adjuvant upon the testis of guinea pigs. *J. Embryol. Exp. Morphol.* 6:94, 1958.

38. Brown P.C., Glynn L.E., Holborow E.J.: The pathogenesis of experimental allergic orchitis in guinea pigs. *J. Pathol.* 86:505, 1963.

39. Bishop D.W., Carlson G.L.: Immunologically induced aspermatogenesis in guinea pigs. *Ann. N.Y. Acad. Sci.* 124:247, 1965.

40. Brown P.C., Glynn L.E.: The early lesion of experimental orchitis in guinea pigs: An immunological correlation. *J. Pathol.* 98:277, 1969.

41. Tung K.S.K., Unanue E.R., Dixon F.J.: The immunopathology of experimental allergic orchitis. *Am. J. Pathol.* 60:313, 1970.

42. Johnson M.H.: Changes of the blood-testis barrier of the guinea pig in relation to histological damage following isoimmunization with testis. *J. Reprod. Fertil.* 22:119, 1970.

43. Bishop D.W.: Aspermatogenesis induced by testicular antigen uncombined with adjuvant. *Proc. Soc. Exp. Biol. Med.* 107:116, 1961.

44. Waksman B.H.: A histologic study of the auto-allergic testis lesion in the guinea pig. *J. Exp. Med.* 109:311, 1959.

45. Johnson M.H.: Physiological mechanisms for the immunological isolation of spermatozoa. *Adv. Reprod. Physiol.* 6:279, 1973.

46. Tung K.S.K., Alexander N.J.: Autoimmune reactions in the testis, in Johnson A. D., Gomes W. R. (eds.): *The Testis,* vol. 4. New York and London, Academic Press, 1977.

47. Pokorna A.: Induction of experimental autoimmune aspermatogenesis by immune serum fractions. *Folia Biol. (Praha)* 16:320, 1970.

48. Voisin G.A., Toullet F.: Etude sur l'orchite aspermatogénétique autoimmune et les autoantigenes des spermatozoides chez le cobaye. *Ann. Inst. Pasteur (Paris)* 81:727, 1968.

49. Willson J.T., Jones N.A., Katsh S.: Induction of aspermatogenesis by transfer of immune sera or cells. *Int. Arch. Allergy Appl. Immunol.* 43: 172, 1972.

50. Rapaport F.T., Sampath A., Kano K., et al.: Immunological effects of thermal injury: I. Inhibition of spermatogenesis in guinea pigs. *J. Exp. Med.* 130:1411, 1969.

51. Fernandez-Collazo E., Thierer E., Mancini R.E.: Immunologic and testicular response in guinea pigs after unilateral thermal orchitis. *J. Allergy Clin. Immunol.* 49:167, 1972.

52. Seidenkranz H.G., Holtz W., Smidt D., et al.: Untersuchungen zum Einfluss von Azathioprin auf Fortpflanzungsfunktionen beim Göttinger Miniaturschwein. *Dtsch. Tierärztl. Wochenschr.* 82:221, 1975.

18 / Technique for Orchiopexy

ERIC W. FONKALSRUD, M.D.

ALTHOUGH SURGICAL PLACEMENT of an undescended testis into the scrotum was first attempted by Rosenmerkel[1] in 1820, and reported occasionally by surgeons during the ensuing years,[2, 3] the results were unsatisfactory and the procedure fell into disrepute until 1899 when Bevan[4] published the results of an improved technique. In his original report, Bevan described the basic principles of testicular mobilization that are fundamental to the modern technique of orchiopexy. The following summary or his original operative technique was compiled by Charney and Wolgin.[5]

"An incision 3 inches long is made over the inguinal canal and the external oblique fascia is divided, as are all the coverings of the cord down to the peritoneum. The vas deferens and spermatic vessels are isolated and separated from the peritoneum for a distance of 2 to 3 inches within the abdomen. The processus vaginalis has been separated from the cord, ligated at the internal inguinal ring, and divided one-half inch below the ligature. All of the coverings of the cord are removed so that the testicle hangs suspended by the vas and spermatic vessels. A large pocket is made in the scrotum by blunt dissection, taking care to open the scrotal neck wide enough to admit only the testis which is then inserted into the pocket. Closure is carried out according to the Bassini technique for repair of inguinal hernia. In addition, the superficial fascia is sutured to the aponeurosis of the external oblique, obliterating the alveolar space between the superficial and deep fascia in front of the external ring, the most likely place for retraction of the testis."

For patients in whom the internal spermatic vessels were too short to permit scrotal placement, Bevan[6] later recommended dividing all the structures of the cord except the vas deferens and its associated deferential artery and vein.

The principle of fixation was combined with Bevan's technique of testicular mobilization by Torek[7] in 1909. The essential features of the

Torek operation consisted of "laying bare the testicle, thinning down the cord till it consists of nothing but vas deferens and spermatic vessels, and continuing the dissection of the vessels upward as far as necessary to allow the testicle to come well down without traction." Torek then recommended incising the lower surface of the scrotum, bringing out the testis and suturing it to the fascia on the inner surface of the thigh. The cut edges of the scrotum were then sutured to the edges of the thigh incision around the testis. After two to three months a second operation was performed to surgically separate the testis and scrotum from the thigh. Ombredanne[8] recommended securing the testis in place by passing it through to the opposite side of the scrotum and closing the septum.

Numerous modifications of the Bevan and Torek orchiopexy techniques have been described over the ensuing years, differing mainly in refinements to improve mobilization of the testis and cord, as well as in methods of fixation. LaRoque,[9] Yodice,[10] Rosenblatt,[11] and others emphasized careful dissection of the retroperitoneal space to mobilize the spermatic artery and vein high enough to permit repositioning of the entire cord in an almost direct line to the scrotum. In order to further facilitate movement of the spermatic vessels toward the midline, Davison[12] and Gessner[13] recommended shifting the cord under the deep epigastric vessels and even advised dividing these structures, thus eliminating a major portion of the inguinal canal. On the basis of cadaver studies, Prentiss and associates[14] calculated the actual increased length of the spermatic vessels achievable by retroperitoneal dissection.

Cabot and Nesbit[15] suggested a more gentle and intermittent traction of the testis than described by Torek. These authors advised attaching a suture to the lower pole of the gonad and bringing it through the lower scrotum where it is fastened by a rubber band to a tape on the inner surface of the thigh until the testis becomes fixed to the scrotal tissues. Gross[16] described a more extensive retroperitoneal dissection mobilizing the spermatic vessels up to the inferior pole of the kidney and the vas deferens down to the base of the bladder, thus moving the cord even closer to the midline. Gross also popularized the one-stage operation by fixing the testis to tape on the contralateral thigh with a traction stitch and rubber band. Subsequent modifications of this procedure have included placing the traction stitch on the gubernaculum rather than on the testis[17] and even leaving the stitch in place for as long as a year.[18] A wide variety of materials has been suggested as the optimal traction stitch, including nylon, catgut, wire, silk, linen, and cotton. Refining the fixation technique by placing the

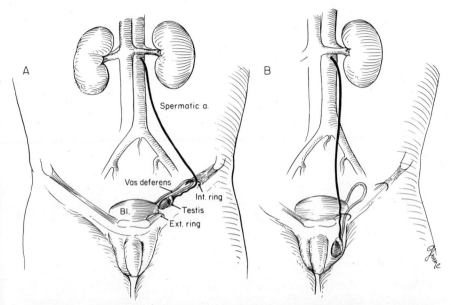

Fig 18–1.—A, lengthy course of spermatic artery descending from aorta through internal inguinal ring to undescended testis in inguinal canal. **B,** by transposing internal inguinal ring medially to pubis, spermatic artery may be lengthened effectively to permit placing testis into scrotum, the basis of standard orchiopexy.[31] (From Fonkalsrud, E.W.: The undescended testis, *Curr. Probl. Surg.* 15:1, 1978. Used with permission.)

testis external to the dartos muscle and internal to the scrotal skin was recommended in 1931 by Petrivalsky[19] and Shoemaker[20]—a method that was repopularized by DeNetto and Goldberg[21] and by Benson and Lofti[22] in 1967 and which is now being used by most pediatric surgeons.

The technique of orchiopexy currently in practice has been described and illustrated by several authors[23-26] with few additional refinements and is shown in the accompanying illustrations. The objective of the repair is to abolish the triangle extending from the renal pedicle to the external inguinal ring with its apex at the internal ring, and to create in its place a direct line from the renal pedicle to the scrotum (Fig 18–1). An incision about 4–6 cm long, slightly larger than that used for inguinal herniorrhaphy, is made through the lowermost abdominal skin crease (Fig 18–2). The external oblique aponeurosis is exposed and opened in the direction of its fibers through the external ring. Occasional patients with high-lying testes will have an unusually small external ring. The testis usually will be found protruding

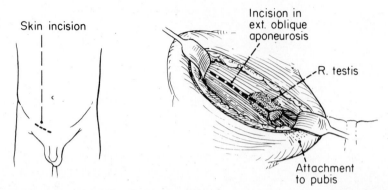

Fig 18–2.—Cutaneous incision for orchiopexy is made through lower abdominal skin crease. External oblique aponeurosis is incised through external ring, exposing testis in its tunica vaginalis, usually located just beneath external ring or in superficial inguinal pouch. (From Fonkalsrud, E.W.: The undescended testis, *Curr. Probl. Surg.* 15:1, 1978. Used with permission.)

through the external ring inferior to the internal oblique muscle with attachments to the pubis.

The testis with its surrounding tunica vaginalis is first mobilized from the gubernaculum and the usually tenacious attachments to the pubis and upper scrotum, permitting it to be elevated with gentle traction (Fig 18–3). The cremaster muscle is freed gently from the sper-

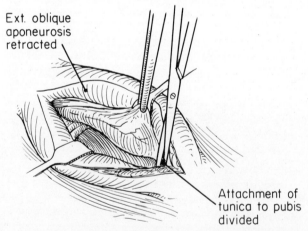

Fig 18–3.—Tunica vaginalis and enclosed testis are mobilized from gubernacular and fascial attachments to pubis and adjacent soft tissues. (From Fonkalsrud, E.W.: The undescended testis, *Curr. Probl. Surg.* 15:1, 1978. Used with permission.)

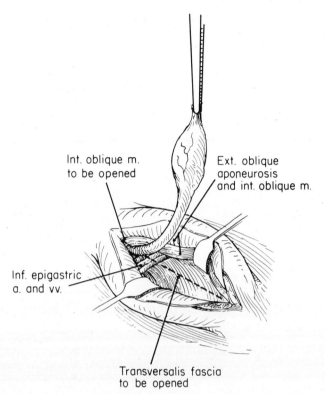

Int. oblique m.
to be opened

Ext. oblique
aponeurosis
and int. oblique m.

Inf. epigastric
a. and vv.

Transversalis fascia
to be opened

Fig 18–4.—Cremaster muscle is teased free from spermatic vessels and vas up to internal inguinal ring. Internal oblique muscle is divided lateral to internal ring over a distance of 1 1/2 cm. Transversalis fascia and inferior epigastric vessels are exposed. (From Fonkalsrud, E.W.: The undescended testis, *Curr. Probl. Surg.* 15:1, 1978. Used with permission.)

matic vessels and the vas deferens up to the level of the internal inguinal ring. The internal oblique muscle is divided lateral to the internal ring over a distance of 1–2 cm to obtain better exposure (Fig 18–4). The inferior epigastric artery and veins are divided, and the transversalis fascia is opened widely through the internal ring to permit wide exposure to the retroperitoneal space (Fig 18–5). The accompanying hernia sac is then separated from the spermatic vessels and the vas, often a very delicate maneuver because the structures are tenaciously adherent and the sac tears easily. This maneuver may be facilitated by injecting a small amount of saline through a 26-gauge needle between the hernia sac and the cord structures, and then gently developing a plane by blunt dissection with a fine clamp (Fig 18–6).[27]

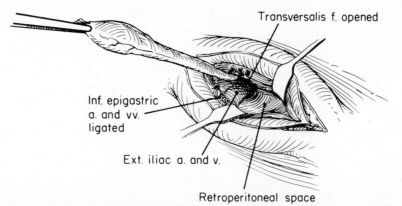

Transversalis f. opened

Inf. epigastric
a. and vv.
ligated

Ext. iliac a. and v.

Retroperitoneal space

Fig 18–5.—Inferior epigastric artery and veins are divided, and transversalis fascia is incised from internal ring medially to pubis to provide wide exposure to retroperitoneal space. Note exposed external iliac vessels. (From Fonkalsrud, E.W.: The undescended testis, *Curr. Probl. Surg.* 15:1, 1978. Used with permission.)

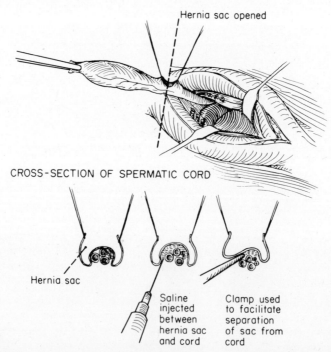

Hernia sac opened

CROSS-SECTION OF SPERMATIC CORD

Hernia sac

Saline
injected
between
hernia sac
and cord

Clamp used
to facilitate
separation
of sac from
cord

Fig 18–6.—Hernia sac is dissected free from spermatic vessels and vas. Cross section shows saline injection technique that occasionally helps to separate delicate but tenaciously adherent hernia sac from spermatic vessels and vas. (From Fonkalsrud, E.W.: The undescended testis, *Curr. Probl. Surg.* 15:1, 1978. Used with permission.)

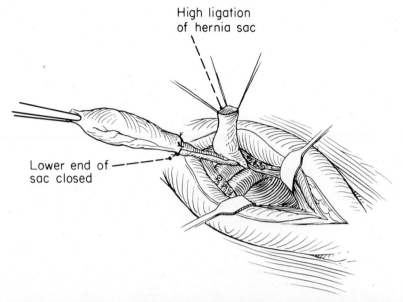

High ligation
of hernia sac

Lower end of
sac closed

Fig 18–7.—Testis is inspected for abnormalities and then replaced in tunica. Biopsy is not routinely performed. Distal end of hernia sac is sutured closed to prevent dislodgment of testis outside tunica. Proximal end of hernia sac is ligated or oversewn and then elevated with posterior peritoneum during subsequent retroperitoneal dissection. (From Fonkalsrud, E.W.: The undescended testis, *Curr. Probl. Surg.* 15:1, 1978. Used with permission.)

A high ligation of the hernia sac is performed with a fine transfixion suture. If the peritoneum tears during this manipulation, it may become necessary to oversew the opening into the peritoneal cavity with a continuous fine suture. The gonad is inspected for size, consistency, and any abnormal features. Biopsy is not routinely recommended, especially in the young child because of the risk of further injury to the delicate organ, unless unusual features are apparent or if the child is past 12 years of age. A thin wedge biopsy running longitudinally on the side opposite the epididymis is the preferred technique, the site being closed with a fine continuous suture. The testis is then replaced into the tunica and the proximal end is closed loosely to prevent dislodgment outside the sac (Fig 18–7). Many surgeons partially remove the tunica; however, caution should be observed to avoid injuring the fine delicate vessels extending to the epididymis and testis, and also to avoid bleeding. Electrocautery is not used during any part of the dissection around the spermatic cord and testis. The dissection is continued into the retroperitoneal space by elevating the peritoneum,

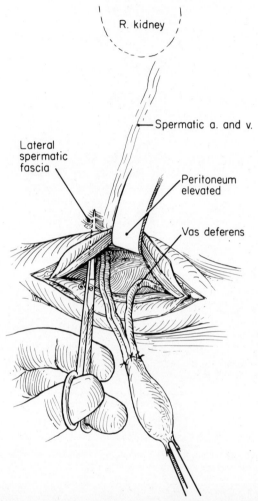

Fig 18–8.—Lateral spermatic fascia is divided, and spermatic vessels are dissected bluntly from posterior surface of peritoneum and retroperitoneal tissues up to lower pole of kidney. (From Fonkalsrud, E.W.: The undescended testis, *Curr. Probl. Surg.* 15:1, 1978. Used with permission.)

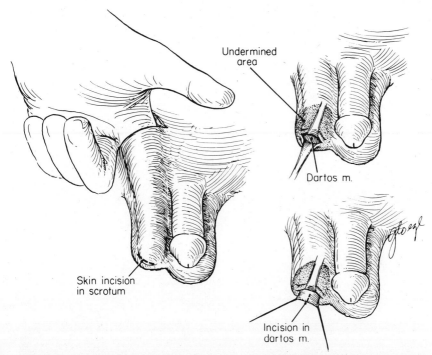

Undermined area

Dartos m.

Skin incision in scrotum

Incision in dartos m.

Fig 18–9.—Scrotum is distended by surgeon's index finger and small incision is made through most dependent portion of scrotal skin. Dartos muscle and fascia are dissected free from scrotal skin to form subcutaneous pouch. (From Fonkalsrud, E. W.: The undescended testis, *Curr. Probl. Surg.* 15:15, 1978. Used with permission.)

sharply dividing the lateral spermatic fascia, and bluntly mobilizing the spermatic vessels up to the lower pole of the kidney and mobilizing the vas over to the bladder (Fig 18–8).

The scrotum is then forcibly stretched by inserting a finger through the wound to the lowest portion of the sac. A small incision is made through the scrotal skin at this point, and a space large enough to easily accommodate the testis is developed between the dartos muscle and the scrotal skin by blunt dissection (Fig 18–9). A small opening is then placed in the dartos fascia and the muscle layer, through which a clamp is passed superiorly to direct the testis downward through the scrotum (Fig 18–10). To permit optimal vascular flow, the spermatic vessels must not be twisted. The upper edge of the tunica is stitched to the dartos layer circumferentially to prevent upward displacement

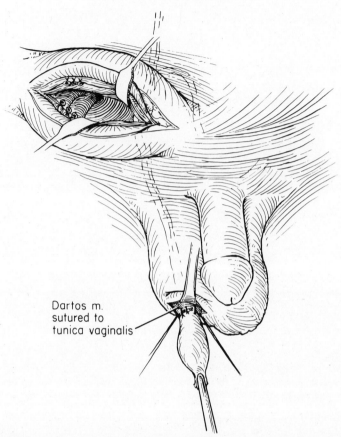

Dartos m.
sutured to
tunica vaginalis

Fig 18–10.—Testis is brought down through opening in dartos muscle and placed in subcutaneous scrotal pouch. Dartos muscle is sutured to upper end of tunica circumferentially to secure gonad in scrotum. (From Fonkalsrud, E.W.: The undescended testis, *Curr. Probl. Surg.* 15:1, 1978. Used with permission.)

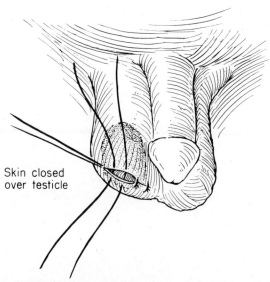

Fig 18–11.—Scrotal skin is closed over testis with absorbable sutures. (From Fonkalsrud, E.W.: The undescended testis, *Curr. Probl. Surg.* 15:1, 1978. Used with permission.)

or subsequent torsion. The scrotal skin is closed loosely with fine absorbable sutures (Fig 18–11). The transversalis fascia is then closed with nonabsorbable sutures, leaving a small opening just lateral to the pubis to function as the new internal inguinal ring (Fig 18–12). The internal oblique muscle is sutured to the shelving edge of the inguinal ligament, again leaving a small opening medially for the new internal ring. The external oblique aponeurosis is approximated, and the skin is closed by the same technique used for herniorrhaphy wounds.

The patient is discharged from the hospital on the second or third postoperative day, depending on his age. Although the external ring is located almost directly over the new internal ring, seemingly conducive to development of a direct hernia, this complication is extremely rare.

In occasional patients with low-lying testes, the spermatic vessels can be mobilized adequately without extensive dissection of the posterior wall of the inguinal canal, and the testis can be secured in the scrotum by the dartos pouch technique or by placing a nylon pull-out stitch secured over a fine gauze roll during five to seven days (Fig 18–13). This technique is particularly helpful in young infants who

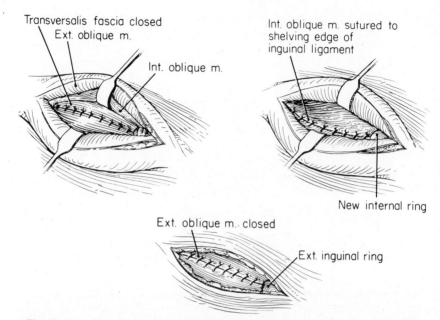

Fig 18–12.—Transversalis fascia is reapproximated, leaving small opening just lateral to pubis to serve as new internal inguinal ring. Internal oblique muscle is approximated to shelving edge of inguinal ligament, again leaving an opening for spermatic cord medially. External oblique aponeurosis is reapproximated. (From Fonkalsrud, E.W.: The undescended testis, *Curr. Probl. Surg.* 15:1, 1978. Used with permission.)

undergo early orchiopexy because of a symptomatic inguinal hernia that requires urgent repair. Experience with this technique has not been entirely satisfactory, particularly if any tension is required to hold the testis in the scrotum, inasmuch as the gonad tends to retract superiorly to the level of the pubis after the pull-out stitch is removed. The dartos pouch method of scrotal attachment is therefore preferred in almost all patients. Careful deliberation should precede the decision to abandon the retroperitoneal dissection portion of the orchiopexy, because, if after operation the gonad retracts upward, a secondary orchiopexy is far more likely to injure the vascular supply to the gonad than does the first operative procedure.

Flinn and King[28] recommended a midline transabdominal approach that is especially useful for patients with bilateral high cryptorchidism because it allows bringing both testes down through a single incision (Fig 18–14). This operation is particularly suitable for patients in

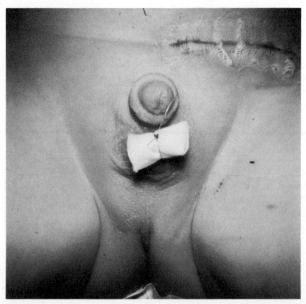

Fig 18–13. — Three-month-old infant with large inguinal hernia and cana-licular undescended testis who underwent urgent herniorrhaphy and simul-taneous orchiopexy. Low-lying testis is held in position for five to seven days by nylon pull-out stitch secured over fine gauze roll. (From Fonkalsrud, E.W.: *Surg. Clin. North Am.* 50:847, 1970. Used with permission.)

whom the inguinal structures have been distorted from previous oper-ations, as well as for those with suspected testicular agenesis or inter-sex malformations, since abdominal exploration may be very helpful in identifying internal genital organs. These authors noted uniformly good results in each of the 25 patients on whom the operation was performed.[28] The preperitoneal approach also has been recommended as a satisfactory method for mobilizing the testis and spermatic cord.[29-31]

Bilateral undescended testes may be repaired under the same anes-thetic without undue risk, if the gonad resides in a low position, e.g., the superficial inguinal pouch. Nevertheless many surgeons prefer to stage repair of bilateral undescent over a period of three to four months in order to minimize tension on the abdominal wall recon-struction.

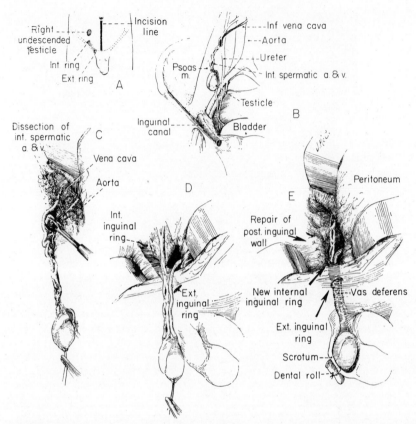

Fig 18–14.–A, midline approach to orchiopexy. **B,** diagrammatic view of intra-abdominal testis. **C,** right testis and cord after complete mobilization. Peritoneum remains intact and is retracted medially. Artery and vein may be dissected to their origins under direct vision. **D,** testis is prepared for placement in scrotum. **E,** completed orchiopexy; spermatic cord traverses abdominal wall immediately lateral to pubic tubercle. (From Flinn and King, *Surg. Gynecol. Obstet.* 131:285, 1971. Used with permission.)

REFERENCES

1. Rosenmerkel J.F.: Ueber die Radicalcur des in der Weiche liegenden Testikels bei nicht Descensus Desselben. Munich, J. Lindauer, 1820.
2. Adams J.E.: Remarks on a case of transition of the testicle into the peritoneum. *Lancet* 1:710, 1871.
3. Schüller M.: On inguinal testicle and its operative treatment by transplantation into the scrotum. *Ann. Anat. Surg.* 4:89, 1881.
4. Bevan A.D.: Operation for undescended testicle and congenital inguinal hernia. *J.A.M.A.* 33:773, 1899.
5. Charney C.W., Wolgin W.: *Cryptorchidism.* New York, Hoeber Medical Division, Harper & Row, 1957.

6. Bevan A.D.: Surgical treatment of undescended testicle: A further contribution. *J.A.M.A.* 41:718, 1903.
7. Torek F.: The technique of orchiopexy. *N.Y. State J. Med.* 90:948, 1909.
8. Ombredanne L.: Sur l'orchiopexie. *Bull. Soc. Pediatr. (Paris)* 25:473, 1927.
9. LaRoque G.P.: A modification of Bevan's operation for undescended testicle. *Ann. Surg.* 94:314, 1931.
10. Yodice A.: Ectopia testicular—su tratamiento por la orquidolisis del valle. *Rev. Med. Latino Am.* 21:757, 1956.
11. Rosenblatt M.S.: Undescended testicle. *Am. J. Surg.* 59:232, 1945.
12. Davison C.: The surgical treatment of undescended testicle. *Surg. Gynecol. Obstet.* 12:283, 1911.
13. Gessner H.B.: Davison's operation for undescended testicle. *New Orleans Med. Surg. J.* 65:641, 1913.
14. Prentiss R.J., Weickgenant C.J., Moses J.J., et al.: Undescended testis: Surgical anatomy of spermatic vessels, spermatic surgical triangles, and lateral spermatic ligament. *J. Urol.* 83:686, 1960.
15. Cabot H., Nesbit R.M.: Undescended testis. *Arch. Surg.* 22:850, 1931.
16. Gross R.E.: *The Surgery of Infancy and Childhood: Its Principles and Techniques.* Philadelphia, W. B. Saunders Co., 1953.
17. Wolfson W.L., Turkeltaub S.M.: A modified Torek operation. *Am. J. Surg.* 25:494, 1934.
18. Ewart E.E.: The technique of orchiopexy. *Surg. Clin. North Am.* 22:851, 1942.
19. Petrivalsky J.: Zur Behandlung des Leistenhoden. *Zentralbl. Chir.* 58:1001, 1939.
20. Shoemaker J.: Uber Cryptorchismus und seine Behandlung. *Chirurg* 4:1, 1932.
21. DeNetto N.F., Goldberg H.M.: A method of orchidopexy. *Surg. Gynecol. Obstet.* 118:840, 1964.
22. Benson C.D., Lofti M.W.: The pouch technique in the surgical correction of cryptorchidism in infants and children. *Surgery* 62:967, 1967.
23. Snyder W.H. Jr., Greaney E.M. Jr.: Cryptorchidism, in Mustard W., Ravitch M.M., Snyder W.H. Jr., et al. (eds.): *Pediatric Surgery,* ed. 2. Chicago, Year Book Medical Publishers, Inc., 1969.
24. Gross R.E., Jewett T.C. Jr.: Surgical experiences from 1,222 operations for undescended testes. *J.A.M.A.* 160:634, 1956.
25. Laughlin V.C.: Orchidofunicolysis. *J. Urol.* 77:39, 1957.
26. Prentiss R.J., Mullenix R.B., Whisenand J.M.: Medical and surgical treatment of cryptorchidism. *Arch. Surg.* 70:283, 1955.
27. Clatworthy H.W. Jr.: Personal communication.
28. Flinn R.A., King L.R.: Experiences with the midline transabdominal approach in orchiopexy. *Surg. Gynecol. Obstet.* 131:285, 1971.
29. Boley S.J., Kleinhaus S.A.: A place for the Cheatle-Henry approach in pediatric surgery. *J. Pediatr. Surg.* 1:394, 1966.
30. Lipton S.: Use of the Cheatle-Henry approach in the treatment of cryptorchidism. *Surgery* 50:846, 1961.
31. Fonkalsrud E.W.: Current concepts in the management of the undescended testis. *Surg. Clin. North Am.* 50:847, 1970.

19 / Management of High Undescended Testis

JAY L. GROSFELD, M.D.

ALTHOUGH ORCHIOPEXY usually is a satisfactory operation for the undescended testis positioned in the lower inguinal canal or in an ectopic location outside the external inguinal ring, management of the high undescended testis remains a formidable clinical problem.[1-3] For years it has been well recognized that the higher the location of the undescended testis, the worse the operative and functional result. In a significant number of children (>20%), the undescended testis resides high in the inguinal canal near the vicinity of the internal inguinal ring or in an intra-abdominal location. In a report concerning more than 700 cases of undescended testis, Cywes[3] reported that 16% occurred high in the canal and 6% were intra-abdominal.

Performance of a standard orchiopexy, with redirection of the vascular pedicle, often fails to shorten the pathway to the scrotum effectively in patients with a high-lying testis. Indeed, a failure rate exceeding 50% has led surgeons to pursue a number of operative alternatives. This chapter will describe the current methods of managing the high undescended testis and recommend a premeditated long-loop vas orchiopexy based on collateral testicular circulation.

PREOPERATIVE EVALUATION

The high undescended testis is often impalpable on examination, and its actual occurrence is difficult to assess even during a carefully performed physical examination. In a review of 3,420 cases of undescended testes, Levitt et al.[1] noted that the testis was impalpable in 694 patients (20%). Although most cases of impalpable testis occur in otherwise normal boys, in some conditions a high testicular location (especially intra-abdominal) is more common. These include instances of prune belly syndrome,[4, 5] Aarskog syndrome,[6, 7] Noonan's syndrome,[8] Lowe's syndrome (cerebro-ocular renal dystrophy), lentigines (Leopard) syndrome, de Lange syndrome, and the trisomy 13–15 and 16–18 syndromes, as well as a number of intersex problems.

In 1969, Ehrlich et al.[9] reported that HCG injections achieved a 16% incidence of descent in patients with unilateral undescended testes. Since that time, this treatment method has been frequently referred to and extensively used by pediatricians. Unfortunately, these data were severely flawed by the retrospective nature of the study, the lack of untreated controls, and the reliance on multiple examiners of the involved children.[10] That 84% of patients failed to improve with this therapy caused serious concern among most pediatric surgeons and urologists. Ehrlich[10] recently has reversed his opinion favoring HCG treatment and has abandoned its use in the unilateral undescended testis. More recent data suggest that synthetic LH-RH given intranasally may produce testicular descent in cryptorchid children (see Chapter 9).[11, 12] This mode of therapy is noninvasive (no injection necessary), is painless, and has no serious androgenic side effects. Cywes[3] reported descent in 11% of children with impalpable testis treated with intranasal LH-RH therapy. Although these observations are encouraging and suggest that this form of therapy may prove useful, the data are derived from a relatively small number of cases and there were no controls. Concise, controlled studies involving a sufficient number of patients to yield statistically significant data are required to evaluate this treatment method.

Occasionally examination under anesthesia immediately before an anticipated operation will eliminate a few cases of retractile testis initially considered impalpable, thus obviating an unnecessary operative procedure. In most cases (>75%), however, the "impalpable" testis can be felt preoperatively near the internal ring under these relaxed conditions. Despite the aid of anesthetic relaxation, however, preoperative examination cannot definitely distinguish between an intra-abdominal testis and monorchism. Although HCG stimulation and measurement of serum testosterone, FSH, and LH levels can distinguish children with bilateral undescended testis from those with probable anorchism (and possibly avoid operation in the latter group), these studies are ineffective in cases of unilateral cryptorchidism and inaccurate in patients beyond 35 years of age.[1, 10, 13]

Preoperative localization of an impalpable testis by herniography has been advocated by White et al.[14]; their success rate was 33% with testes found in an intracanalicular location. This study (which has an 11% complication rate), however, failed to distinguish cases of monorchism from intra-abdominal testis and probably unnecessarily exposed the involved children to radiation. Transfemoral selective arteriography also has been suggested as a diagnostic adjunct for high undescended testes.[15, 16] Angiography may require a general anesthetic and the results have been inconsistent. Spermatic venography has been recommended by Glickman et al.[17] and Amin and Wheeler[18] to localize the impalpable testis in order to expedite surgical therapy. In this method, identification of a vein that terminates in a pampiniform-like plexus usually signals the presence of a testis. This procedure is more readily performed on the left side where the spermatic vein empties into the left renal vein. However, because high undescended testes are found easily at operation near the internal ring either in the inguinal canal or intra-abdominally, venograms usually are unnecessary.[1] Therefore, we do not perform this test routinely but might consider it in the rare instance when an inguinal, retroperitoneal, and/or intraperitoneal exploration fails to locate the testis or a blind-ending spermatic vessel. Moreover failure to demonstrate an internal spermatic vein on venography would suggest an absent testis (4% of cases).[1]

Although radioisotopic scans, ultrasonography, and CAT have been suggested as adjunctive diagnostic tests for localizing the high undescended testis, such studies are rarely indicated and not routinely recommended.

SURGICAL CONSIDERATIONS

The goal of surgical therapy for the high undescended testis is to place the testis in a normal intrascrotal location to allow appropriate germinal cell growth, improve the chance for fertility, assuage potential psychologic trauma associated with a single testis, and reduce the risk of malignancy (especially for intra-abdominal testis) in later life. Current popular methods of surgical therapy for high undescended testes include (1) standard or transabdominal staged orchiopexy, (2) long-loop vas operation based on testicular collateral circulation, (3) microvascular surgery, and (4) orchiectomy with prosthetic replacement in selected cases.

Exploration should be done initially through a transverse inguinal wound inasmuch as 75–80% of high undescended testes are located near the internal inguinal ring. Failure to find the testis in these typical locations does not necessarily indicate a diagnosis of testicular agenesis, however, and therefore a formal abdominal exploration should be undertaken. Similarly, the finding of a blind-ending vas deferens with or without associated epididymal tissues does not confirm testicular absence, because the embryologic origin of the gonads and the ductal tissues is separate, and these structures may be some distance apart.[1, 19, 20] This finding may occur in as high as 11% of cases and should prompt a diligent search for testicular tissue. On the other hand, the discovery of a blind-ending spermatic vessel is a good indication of an absent testis and thus no further exploration is warranted.[1] In most cases, however, a testis is located and orchiopexy should be attempted. Boys with intracanalicular undescended testis usually have an associated patent processus vaginalis or an overt clinical hernia sac, which should be separated and high ligation done by suture fixation at the level of the internal ring during orchiopexy.

STAGED ORCHIOPEXY

Persky and Albert[21] advised the use of a staged procedure for patients with high undescended testes. Using the standard orchiopexy techniques described in the previous chapter, the testis was mobilized, the vas deferens and spermatic vessels were preserved, and the peritoneal bands freed high into the retroperitoneal space to the level of the lower pole of the kidney. During the first-stage procedure, the testis was attached to the external inguinal ring or pubis by suture fixation. These authors reported that no discomfort or injury to the testis was noted in their patients.[21] A second-stage procedure was then performed between eight and 16 months later. A careful redissection of the tissues off the cord vessels was done, which was difficult in the presence of fibrous adhesions. This technique was successful in allowing the testis to be brought down ultimately to an intrascrotal location and fixed with a subdartos technique in two thirds of cases. In one third of these boys, however, this procedure failed, and an orchiectomy had to be performed. Incision of the lateral spermatic fascia and the transversalis fascia medially allows better mobilization of the testis and its vessels. Division of the epigastric vessels then enables the testis and spermatic vessels to be redirected and gains some length (Fig 19–1). Unfortunately, this maneuver, which is so useful for testes residing in the lower end of the inguinal canal, often does not allow the testis, when in higher locations, sufficient length to reach the scrotal sac.

Corkery[22] described a technique to protect the testis and its vessels at the first-stage operation by temporarily encasing these structures in Silastic sheeting to prevent scarring (Fig 19–2). This allows a safer second-stage procedure by preventing adherence of the testes, vas, and spermatic vessels to surrounding tissues. Nevertheless, the re-

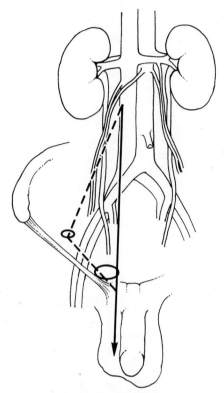

Fig 19–1.—Illustration demonstrating that redirecting testis in a straight line medially increases length of spermatic vessels.

sults of this technique vary considerably and usually depend on the surgeon's skill and an assessment of the subsequent size, consistency, and mobility of the fixated testis compared to its normally descended counterpart. Firor[23] reported success in 30 of 32 boys with staged procedures and Zer et al.[24] in 77% (48/62) with intra-abdominal testes who underwent operations. In a careful review concerning staged orchiopexy, however, Redman[25] observed that elongation of the spermatic cord by surgical manipulation had not been documented and suggested that the good results reported by proponents of staged orchiopexy were due to an inadequately performed initial operation and that they also lacked long-term data.

The patient's age may affect the ability of the surgeon to perform a more standard orchiopexy procedure for intra-abdominal testes. In infants with prune belly syndrome, Woodard and Parrott[5] were able to perform a trans-abdominal single-stage orchiopexy. In these infants the testis was found overlying the ureters low in the pelvis. By mobi-

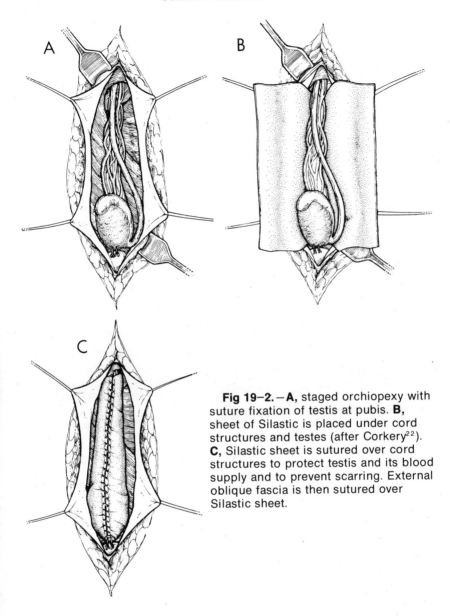

Fig 19–2. — **A,** staged orchiopexy with suture fixation of testis at pubis. **B,** sheet of Silastic is placed under cord structures and testes (after Corkery[22]). **C,** Silastic sheet is sutured over cord structures to protect testis and its blood supply and to prevent scarring. External oblique fascia is then sutured over Silastic sheet.

lizing and straightening the dilated and tortuous ureters, these authors mobilized the spermatic vessels cephalad to the lower pole of the kidney to achieve significant length. The testis was then placed into the scrotum by a transabdominal approach, perforating the medial wall of the inguinal canal at the pubic tubercle (i.e., near the external ingui-

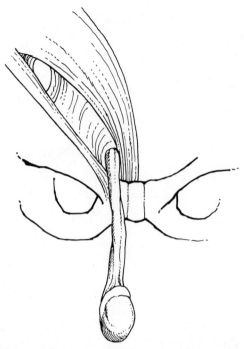

Fig 19–3.—Illustration of exit site of testis over pubis.

nal ring) (Fig 19–3). However, these authors could not achieve the same results in older children; they noted that the first stage often retracts and that a second-stage procedure might be necessary.[5] In their report, a good result in cases of bilateral undescended testes was the presence of *one* scrotal testis without atrophy on anatomical assessment.[5] Inasmuch as paternity has not been reported in prune belly patients and few data are available concerning semen analysis, the actual functional status following such procedures is yet to be determined.

LONG-LOOP VAS ORCHIOPEXY

The modern era long-loop vas orchiopexy was described in 1959 by Fowler and Stephens,[26] who observed that in patients with high undescended testes, the vas deferens often was elongated, extending down (frequently through the external ring) well below the high-lying gonad and then looping back to rejoin the testis. The testicular vessels are short, but the vas deferens and its companion vessels are long. This secondary vascular loop develops from the vessels of the vas deferens, the collaterals arising from the deep epigastric vessels, and

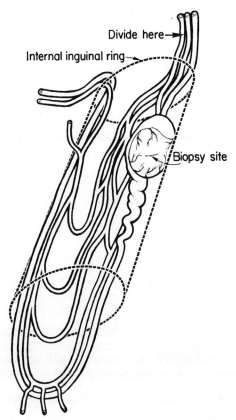

Divide here→

Internal inguinal ring

Biopsy site

Fig 19–4. — Illustration of long-loop vas variant of high undescended testis located near internal inguinal ring. If collateral circulation from vas deferens and gubernaculum is adequate, main vascular pedicle may be ligated high above testis.

myriad branches entering the posterior wall of the processus vaginalis from the area of the gubernaculum testis (Fig 19–4). This vascular network results in a rich collateral testicular circulation even though the testis remains fixed in a high-lying position. Under such anatomical conditions, high ligation and division of the main vascular pedicle to the testis may be feasible, allowing the testis to be placed in an intrascrotal position.[2, 26]

OPERATIVE TECHNIQUE

A transverse skin and subcutaneous fascial incision is made in the inguinal crease over the inguinal canal. The inguinal ligament and external inguinal ring are exposed, and the external oblique fascia is opened perpendicular to the ring in the long axis of its fibers. The cremasteric muscle and fascia are separated. The anteromedial hernia sac is identified and the level of the undescended testis noted. A low position of the vas deferens is seen looping down the posterior medial wall of the sac and returning upward to the epididymis and testis. The hernia sac is then opened and dissected from the testicular vessels well above the gonad, and the neck of the hernia sac is suture ligated with 4–0 or 3–0 silk (Fig 19–5, A). The collateral circulation to the testis is checked by placing a small vascular (bulldog) clamp high on the major spermatic pedicle one to two inches above the testis. A small incision is made in the tunica albuginea to observe the area for bright red bleeding. If brisk bleeding continues from the cut surface of the testis for three or four minutes, the collateral circulation is considered adequate and the major spermatic vascular pedicle is then doubly ligated with 3–0 silk and divided above the level of the occluding clamp (Fig 19–5, B).

The vascular anastomotic arcade is identified between the vas deferens and testicular vessels running marginal to the epididymis. By careful dissection aided by transillumination of the cord structures (with a portable sterile light or a headlight and ×2.5 to ×3 magnifying loupes), the long-loop vas and its vascular arcade can be lengthened by incising between the two limbs of the vascular loop. Division of as few of the small vascular arcades as necessary to permit placing the testis in the scrotal sac is accomplished. The distal posterior wall of the residual hernia sac should be left attached to the testis, since collaterals from the gubernaculum also may extend to the testis. The testis is placed in the scrotum and carefully fixed in a subdartos location under direct vision via a small incision in the scrotum (Fig 19–5, C through H).

Moschowitz[27] initially described the long-loop vas variant in children with undescended testis in 1910. Fowler and Stephens[26] reported using this technique in 12 patients with undescended testes, obtaining a good result in eight. Biopsy done in four of these testes showed that histologically the Leydig cells survived interruption of the major vascular pedicle. Nunn and Stephens[4] subsequently reported that in boys with prune belly syndrome, two-thirds had adequate testosterone levels following long-loop vas orchiopexy. Barnhouse[28] similarly reported successful long-loop vas orchiopexy in three children with prune belly syndrome and intra-abdominal testes. Brendler and Wulfson[29] described five successful cases of the long-loop vas procedure and stressed two points: (1) absolutely no dissection should be performed within the substance of the cord; and (2) anastomotic vessels may join with the main spermatic trunk at some distance above the testis, and therefore division of the vessels must be done well above the testis.

Clatworthy, et al.[2] described 32 long-loop vas procedures in 27 boys with cryptorchidism (bilateral in five). The ages of the patients ranged from two to 18 years; however, age did not predict the anatomical outcome of the procedure. Biopsies from children older than five years tended to show histologic abnormalities. Based on more recent histological and ultrastructural data (see Chapter 16), the current recommended age for orchiopexy at our hospital is two years.

The best results are achieved when the long-loop vas orchiopexy procedure is premeditated. To achieve success with this operation, it is essential that the collateral blood supply remain intact. The posterior wall of the hernia sac proximal to the testis and epididymis must not be mobilized; the floor of the inguinal canal and the deep epigastric vessels must remain undisturbed. If a standard orchiopexy dissection is initially attempted, most or all of the collateral circulation to the testis is destroyed, and dividing the main spermatic vessels as an afterthought has a disastrous outcome with an atrophic testis. Previously reported poor results from this procedure may have been related to extensive dissection of the cord and inguinal canal performed prior to vessel ligation. In 21 patients (including 14 boys with intra-abdominal testes) in whom a long-loop vas orchiopexy was premeditated, a good result, judged by scrotal position and normal size for age, was obtained in 18 cases (86%) (Table 19–1).[2]

Two types of cryptorchid testes are anatomically unsuited for a long-loop vas orchiopexy: (1) the testis with a very short vas deferens as well as short spermatic vessels, and (2) the hypoplastic-appearing testis in which it is uncertain that adequate vascular anastomoses are present.

Prospects are often dismal for boys with a clinically impalpable testis; however, in those with the long-loop vas anatomical variant of undescended testis, this procedure is an extremely simple one-stage procedure. When done on a premeditated basis, it effectively salvages the testis in most cases (86%). The long-loop vas procedure is obviously an improvement over multistaged procedures or orchiectomy, and we prefer it for patients with an appropriate anatomical condition.

MICROVASCULAR PROCEDURES

Inasmuch as the results of orchiopexy for high undescended testis have been unsuccessful when standard and staged forms of orchio-

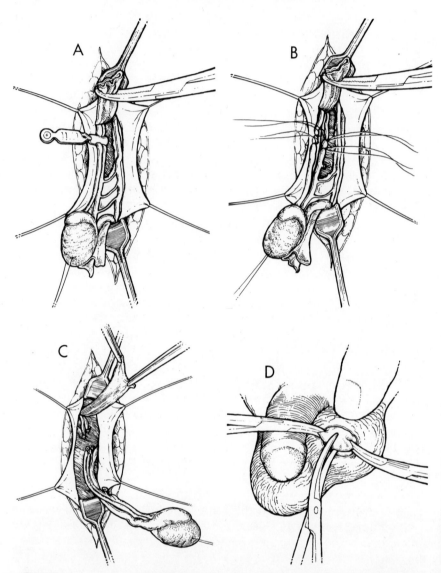

Fig 19–5. – **A,** associated hernia sac is dissected high at internal ring. Small bulldog clamp is placed well above gonad (1–2 inches). If brisk bleeding occurs from small incision in tunica, collateral circulation is adequate. **B,** main vascular pedicle is tied in continuity with 3–0 silk above level of vascular clamp and divided. **C,** ligation and division of most superior collateral vessel from vas deferens to gain appropriate length for testis to reach scrotum. **D,** fingertip dissection makes pouch in previously unused scrotal sac. Incision is made and dartos muscle is incised. *(Continued)*

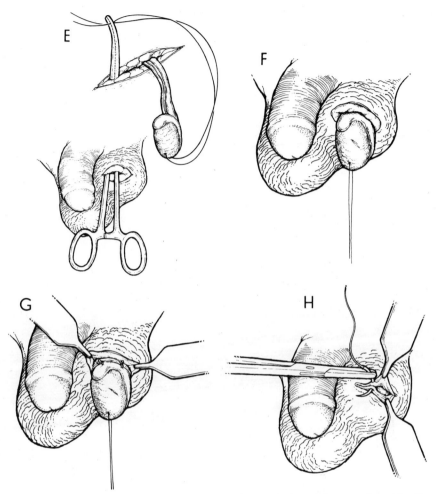

Fig 19–5 (cont).—**E** and **F,** Kelly clamp is passed up into canal and testis is brought into scrotum. **G** and **H,** testis is fixed to dartos muscle pouch with 4–0 chromic catgut and skin is closed with subcuticular 4–0 plain catgut suture and sealed with collodion.

pexy were performed, attempts have been made to autotransplant a testis at these high sites by microvascular techniques. MacMahon et al.[30] described the use of pudendal or inferior epigastric vessels for this purpose and employed 10–0 monofilament suture material successfully in nine of 10 procedures in laboratory animals. Silber and Kelly[31] as well as Janecka and Romas[32] reported successful clinical microvascular procedures in one and three patients, respectively.

TABLE 19-1.—RESULTS:
PREMEDITATED LONG-LOOP VAS
ORCHIOPEXY (21 CASES)

AGE (Yr)	LOCATION OF TESTIS	RESULTS°
2	Intra-abdominal	Good
3	Intra-abdominal	Good
3	Intra-abdominal	Atrophic at 2 yr
5	Intra-abdominal	Good
5	High canal	Good
5	High canal	Good
5	Intra-abdominal	Good
5	High canal	Good
6	Intra-abdominal	Good
6	Intra-abdominal	Good
7	Intra-abdominal	Good
8	High canal	Good
9	High canal	Good
10	Intra-abdominal	Atrophic at 2 mo
10	Intra-abdominal	Good
10	Intra-abdominal	Poor position
11	High canal	Good
12	Intra-abdominal	Good
15	Intra-abdominal	Good
15	High canal	Good
17	Intra-abdominal	Good

°18 of 21 cases were successful when procedure was done on a premeditated basis (revised after Clatworthy et al.[2]).

This technique may ultimately reduce the need for orchiectomy in selected cases. These procedures will be discussed in more detail in Chapter 23.

THE ROLE OF ORCHIECTOMY

At the time of testicular exploration, if the testis is obviously atrophic (especially in the postpuberal patient with unilateral undescended testis), orchiectomy should probably be performed. This is particularly important in cases of retained intra-abdominal testis, which carry the highest risk of later malignant degeneration. After removal of the testis, a testicular prosthesis should be inserted. Details concerning the atrophic testis and the techniques for prosthetic insertion are presented in depth in Chapter 20.

SUMMARY

A high undescended testis is observed in about 20% of patients with cryptorchid testis. In many of these instances, the testis cannot be palpated. Endocrine tests, angiographic studies (arteriography, venography), or herniograms are not routinely recommended for patients with impalpable unilateral undescended testis. All of these patients require exploration. The high undescended testis will be found in the inguinal canal near the internal ring or in the retroperitoneal space in most cases. At the time of exploration, if a long-loop vas is observed, we believe that a premeditated long-loop vas orchiopexy is the procedure of choice. In other situations, a staged orchiopexy should be attempted and may be easier to perform in a child early in infancy. Finding a blind-ending vas or epididymis at the time of inguinal exploration suggests that the testis may be separate from these structures and usually can be found in a retroperitoneal or intraperitoneal location. On the other hand, identification of blind-ending spermatic vessels indicates monorchism. In boys (especially postpuberal) with unilateral atrophic testis, orchiectomy and prosthetic insertion should be performed.

REFERENCES
1. Levitt S.B., Kogan S.J., Engel R.M., et al.: The impalpable testis: A rational approach to management. *J. Urol.* 120:515, 1978.
2. Clatworthy H.W. Jr., Hollabaugh R., Grosfeld J.L.: The "long-loop-vas" orchidopexy for the high undescended testis. *Am. Surg.* 38:69, 1972.
3. Cywes S.: Undescended testis. Symposium on long-term follow-up in congenital anomalies. Pittsburgh Children's Hospital, Pittsburgh, Oct. 1979.
4. Nunn L.N., Stephens F.D.: The triad syndrome: A composite anomaly of the abdominal wall, urinary system, and testis. *J. Urol.* 86:782, 1961.
5. Woodard J.R., Parrott T.S.: Orchiopexy in the prune-belly syndrome. *Br. J. Surg.* 50:348, 1978.
6. Aarskog D.: A familial syndrome of short stature associated with facial dysplasia and genital anomalies. *J. Pediatr.* 77:856, 1970.
7. Andrassy R.J., Murthy S., Woolley M.M.: Aarskog syndrome: Significance for the surgeon. *J. Pediatr. Surg.* 14:462, 1979.
8. Char F., Rodriguez-Fernandez H.L., Scott C.I.: The Noonan syndrome: A clinical study of 45 cases. *Birth Defects* 8:110, 1972.
9. Ehrlich R.M., Dougherty L.J., Tomasheffsky T., et al.: Effect of gonadotropin in cryptorchidism. *J. Urol.* 102:793, 1969.
10. Ehrlich R.M.: The cryptorchid testis. *Dialogues Pediatr. Urol.* 1(5):6, 1978.
11. Pirazzoli P., Zappula F., Bernardi F., et al.: Luteinizing hormone-releasing hormone nasal spray as therapy for undescended testes. *Arch. Dis. Child.* 53:235, 1978.
12. White M.C., Ginsberg J.: Treatment of cryptorchidism by synthetic luteinizing hormone. *Lancet* 2:1361, 1977.
13. Levitt S.B., Kogan S.J., Schneider K.M.: Endocrine tests in phenotypic children with bilateral impalpable testes can reliably predict "congenital" anorchism. *Urology* 11:11, 1978.

14. White J.J., Haller J.A. Jr., Dorst J.P.: Congenital inguinal hernia and herniography. *Surg. Clin. North Am.* 50:823, 1970.
15. Nordmark L.: Angiography of the testicular artery: I. Method of examination. *Acta Radiol. [Diag.] (Stockh.)* 18:25, 1977.
16. Vitale P.J., Khademi M., Seebode J.J.: Selective gonadal angiography for testicular localization in patients with cryptorchidism. *Surg. Forum* 25: 538, 1974.
17. Glickman M.G., Weiss R. M., Itzchak Y.: Testicular venography for undescended testes. *Am. J. Roentgenol.* 129:67, 1977.
18. Amin M., Wheeler C.S.: Selective testicular venography in abdominal cryptorchidism. *J. Urol.* 115:760, 1976.
19. Nowak K.: Failure of fusion of epididymis and testicle with complete separation of the vas deferens. *J. Pediatr. Surg.* 7:715, 1972.
20. Brothers L.R. III, Weber C.H. Jr., Ball T.P. Jr.: Anorchism vs. cryptorchidism: The importance of a diligent search for an intra-abdominal testis. *J. Urol.* 119:707, 1978.
21. Persky L., Albert D.J.: Staged orchiopexy. *Surg. Gynecol. Obstet.* 132:43, 1971.
22. Corkery J.J.: Staged orchiopexy—a new technique. *J. Pediatr. Surg.* 10: 515, 1975.
23. Firor H.V.: Two-stage orchiopexy. *Arch. Surg.* 102:598, 1971.
24. Zer M., Wolloch Y., Dintsman M.: Staged orchiorrhaphy: Therapeutic procedure in cryptorchic testicle with a short spermatic cord. *Arch. Surg.* 110:387, 1975.
25. Redman J.F.: The staged orchiopexy: A critical review of the literature. *J. Urol.* 117:113, 1977.
26. Fowler R., Stephens F.D.: The role of testicular vascular anatomy in the salvage of the high undescended testis. *Aust. N.Z. J. Surg.* 29:92, 1959.
27. Moschowitz A.V.: The anatomy and treatment of the undescended testis. *Ann. Surg.* 52:821, 1910.
28. Barnhouse D.H.: Prune-belly syndrome. *Br. J. Urol.* 44:356, 1972.
29. Brendler H., Wulfson M.A.: Surgical treatment of the high undescended testis. *Surg. Gynecol. Obstet.* 124:605, 1967.
30. MacMahon R.A., O'Brien B.M., Cussen L.J.: The use of microsurgery in the treatment of the undescended testis. *J. Pediatr. Surg.* 11:52, 1976.
31. Silber S.J., Kelly J.: Successful autotransplantation of an intra-abdominal testis to the scrotum by microvascular technique. *J. Urol.* 115:452, 1976.
32. Janecka I.P., Romas N.A.: Microvascular free transfer of human testes. *J. Plast. Reconstr. Surg.* 63:42, 1979.

20 / Management of Bilateral Undescent and Atrophic Testes

JAY L. GROSFELD, M.D.

CHILDREN WITH BILATERAL undescended testes have unique problems and require careful evaluation with regard to treatment. The incidence of unilateral cryptorchid testis is about one in 150 to 200 boys, whereas in contrast bilateral undescended testes occur in one in 600 boys, and anorchism is found in one in 5,000. Table 20–1 lists six reports concerning children with undescended testes. Of 2,336 cases of undescended testes, 553 (23.6%) were bilateral.[1-6]

More than 6% of boys with bilateral undescended testes have underlying endocrine disorders that may result in hypogonadism.[7] These include hypopituitarism, germinal cell aplasia, Klinefelter's syndrome (XXY), and a variety of intersexual problems with ambiguous genitalia. In patients suspected of having one of these conditions, an early workup should include the following tests:

1. Buccal smear
2. Y chromosome fluorescence
3. Chromosomal karyotype (46 XY)
4. Retrograde urethrography to explore for the presence of a utricular remnant.
5. Intravenous pyelogram

Bilateral undescended testes also are more frequently seen in boys with the prune belly syndrome, Aarskog syndrome, Noonan's syndrome, and hypospadias and in some babies with bladder exstrophy and abdominal wall defects (e.g., gastroschisis, omphalocele).[8]

In boys with bilateral impalpable testes, it is important to distinguish between those with anorchism and those with true bilateral undescent. Gross and Jewett[3] observed a 0.6% incidence of anorchism, noting six cases in 988 boys with cryptorchid testes. A similar incidence was observed by Aynsley-Green et al.[9]

Administration of HCG to males with bilateral impalpable testes

TABLE 20–1.—COMPOSITE SERIES OF
CRYPTORCHID BOYS

AUTHOR	ALL CASES	NO. OF CASES BILATERAL UNDESCENT	% BILATERAL UNDESCENT
Benson and Lofti[1]	332	39	12%
Cywes[2]	769	202	26%
Gross and Jewett[3]	942	241	26%
Hortling et al.[4]	93	33	35%
Sudmann[5]	64	17	26%
Woolley[6]	136	21	15%
Total	2,336	553	(23.3%)

usually can accurately predict that testicular tissue is present and in some cases may induce partial descent to allow gonadal palpation. Lee et al.[10] noted an increased serum level of LH and FSH in males with bilateral anorchism. An elevated FSH level was considered an indicator of compromised testicular function, whereas an elevated LH level was consistent with the presence of atrophic gonadal tissue. Bramble et al.[11] observed an increased serum FSH level in patients with repaired bilateral undescended testes who had severe seminiferous tubule damage. Cywes[2] found an inverse correlation between FSH levels and the mean number of spermatogonia.

Rivarola et al.[12] recommended a trial course of HCG for all patients with nonpalpable testes, in addition to a careful monitoring of plasma testosterone level in boys with testes (even when hypoplastic); however, no changes from baseline testosterone levels were observed in cases of anorchism. Levitt et al.[13] suggested that normal basal HCG, LH, and FSH levels—and an appropriate increase in serum testosterone level over basal values after a challenge with exogenous HCG—indicated that functioning testicular tissue was present and mandated a thorough operative exploration for undescended testes. On the other hand, if the basal FSH and LH levels were elevated, in association with a failure of testosterone levels to increase over basal levels after an HCG challenge, these elevations would be consistent with an absence of functioning testicular tissue. The latter findings in a normal phenotypic male without palpable müllerian structures on rectal examination indicate that the patient has anorchism and therefore no surgical exploration is required. Bilateral or "congenital" anorchism probably is related to a vascular accident (perhaps torsion) that has caused atrophy and resorption of both testes and is sometimes referred to as the vanishing testis syndrome.[8, 14]

Jimenez et al.[15] suggest measuring the serum testosterone level after administering 2,000 IU of HCG daily for three days. If the testosterone level increases, testicular tissue is present. If no increase in testosterone level is noted, a second test dose of 4,000 IU of HCG is given. If no increase in serum testosterone level occurs, a diagnosis of anorchism is made.

In patients with bilateral undescent in whom the testes are palpable, HCG also may be given in an attempt to stimulate descent. Ehrlich et al.[16] observed that a short course of HCG (3,300 IU daily for three days) achieved a 33% rate of bilateral descent. In boys under five years of age, descent was observed in 55% of cases. Human chorionic gonadotropin will cause an increase in spermatic vascular flow and in vessel and testicular size and may facilitate subsequent surgical exploration.[8] Although HCG is now rarely used for treatment of unilateral undescended testes in most children's centers, this therapy may have a role in cases of bilateral undescent when the gonads are palpable, and especially when they are impalpable to rule out anorchism.

OPERATIVE TREATMENT

Exploration is accomplished via a transverse inguinal crease incision. In instances of bilateral undescent in which the testes are palpable within the inguinal canal, a standard orchiopexy procedure, with incision of the lateral spermatic fascia and medial transversalis fascia, and high dissection and redirection of the vascular pedicle, as previously discussed (see Chapters 18 and 19), usually will allow satisfactory placement of the testes in the scrotal sac. A dartos pouch fixation procedure will prevent subsequent retraction. High suture ligation of an accompanying hernia sac or patent processus vaginalis should be done at the level of the internal ring. The procedure also may be performed through an alternative incision, a single transverse (Pfannenstiel) approach to both inguinal areas, as suggested by Levitt et al.[7]

If the testes are found in a high location (e.g., near the internal ring or in the retroperitoneal space), various operative alternatives are available, including transabdominal, staged, and long-loop vas orchiopexy (see Chapter 19). A preperitoneal approach also has been recommended for cases of high bilateral undescended testes.[17, 18]

As previously noted, the premeditated long-loop vas orchiopexy is our procedure of choice when appropriate anatomical considerations prevail.[19] Barnhouse,[20] using the long-loop vas procedure, similarly reported successful bilateral orchiopexy in four patients with the prune belly syndrome.

In patients with the prune belly syndrome, bilateral orchiopexy appears to be more successfully accomplished in infancy than later in childhood. Woodard and Parrott[21] observed that the testes usually were found low in the pelvis overlying the ureters. Ureteral mobilization enabled elongation of the spermatic vessels sufficient to allow the testis to reach the scrotum through a perforation in the medial wall of the inguinal canal at the pubic tubercle. However, these authors reported that retraction of the testis may occur and a second-stage procedure may be required.[21] Their assessment of a successful result for bilateral undescended testes was the presence on physical examination of *one* scrotal testis without atrophy.

Although most authors suggest orchiectomy as the procedure of choice for teenagers with an undescended testis because of the unlikely chance of fertility and the greater risk of malignancy (especially for intra-abdominal testis), in instances of bilateral undescent the testis should probably be preserved for its endocrine effect.[7] These patients should be carefully observed on a long-term basis for possible testicular malignancy.

RESULTS: BILATERAL UNDESCENDED TESTES

In the past a good result following orchiopexy often has been based on an anatomical assessment on physical examination. The size, consistency, and mobility of the testis were used as evaluable criteria. In addition, the scrotal position of the testes (high or low) as well as the histologic appearance of the involved testis also was considered. Moreover paternity, in the past always considered as synonymous with fertility, is not an absolutely accurate method of determining spermatogenic function.

Using anatomical, histologic, and paternity considerations as a guide, Gross and Jewett[3] reported a 79% fertility rate among boys with bilateral undescended testes. Bramble et al.[11] and Scott[22] reported a far lower 48% fertility rate.

More recent data strongly suggest that semen density analysis (sperm count) is the best indicator of fertility.[23] Cywes[2] reported a comparative evaluation of 29 patients with bilateral undescent using anatomical assessment, histologic appearance, and semen analysis as criteria. Ninety percent of patients had a good anatomical result, 75% were histologically acceptable, but only 34% were deemed capable of paternity on the basis of semen analysis. This assessment of testicular function after bilateral orchiopexy clearly indicates that poor histologic results may accompany what is considered a good anatomical result.

TABLE 20–2. – UNDESCENDED
TESTIS: EVALUATION OF
SEMEN ANALYSIS

TESTICULAR STATUS	SPERM COUNT
Good	>60 million/ml
Fair	20–40 million/ml*
Poor	<20 million/ml†

*For borderline cases, sperm morphology and motility are considered.
†Sperm volume <5 cc also considered poor.

Similarly, a deficiency in seminal fluid may be associated with a pathologist's confirmation of good histologic results (Table 20–2).

Using the strict criterion of semen analysis as a guide to fertility in bilateral undescended testes, Cywes[2] suggested that only 10% of cases had semen of good quality and were fully fertile, 23% were fair and might be fertile, and 66% had such poor sperm quality that they were probably sterile. By comparison, similar studies in patients with unilateral undescended testis showed that only 4% were considered sterile (poor), 28% were rated fair, and 68% were probably fertile.[2]

In view of these more recent findings, Jewett[24] reevaluated the data originally presented by Gross and Jewett[3] in 1947. When the material was subjected to stricter criteria, the probable fertility rate was calculated to be a more realistic 38%.

ATROPHIC TESTIS

In patients with a unilateral undescended testis that is obviously atrophic, an orchiectomy should be performed. This is especially urged as the treatment of choice for boys who are not explored until their teens and for those with an atrophic intra-abdominal gonad, inasmuch as this carries the highest probability of subsequent malignancy. In cases of bilateral undescent with atrophic testes, the gonads probably should be retained and brought down to a site where they can be periodically evaluated. The patient and his parents must be carefully advised regarding the risk of malignancy and the fact that the chance for fertility is extremely low (10%). However, it should be explained that this will also preserve some androgenic function for the child.

In patients in whom orchiectomy is performed, as in those with monorchism or anorchism, a testicular prosthesis should be inserted.

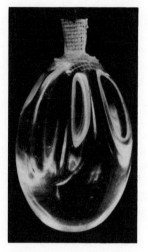

Fig 20–1.—Photograph of Silastic gel-filled testicular prosthesis currently in use.

This cosmetic improvement will prevent or reduce psychologic problems associated with an empty scrotum. The most effective prosthetic replacement is a soft, seamless, ovoid Silastic gonad filled with a silicone gel material,* as advocated by Lattimer et al.[25] (Fig 20 – 1). It comes in four sizes: child, youth, average adult, and large (Table 20 – 3). The prosthetic testis can be resterilized in an autoclave but should not be treated with ethylene oxide, which may cause an adverse tissue reaction.

Contraindications to the use of this prosthesis include an active scrotal infection, history of a recent scrotal infection, or an incomplete or totally undeveloped scrotal sac. The child-size prosthesis is too large for use in infants and toddlers.

TECHNIQUE OF INSERTION

The operative method for inserting the testicular prosthesis depends on when the prosthesis is to be inserted: at the time of orchiectomy or at a later date. In the former situation, the empty scrotal sac is stretched by finger dissection through the inguinal incision. A moist sponge is temporarily packed firmly into the scrotal sac to maintain the previously stretched area. In instances of unilateral atrophic undescended testis or monorchism, the normal testis is an appropriate guide to determine the size of the testicular prosthesis. The sharp edges of the dacron tab used to suture the prosthesis in place are

---

*Dow-Corning Co., Midland, Michigan.

TABLE 20-3.—SILASTIC GEL
TESTICULAR PROSTHESIS

SIZE	DIMENSIONS (cm)	GEL VOL. (cc)
Child	2.0×2.5	5.3
Youth	2.4×3.4	9.4
Average adult	2.8×4.2	16.2
Large	3.0×4.7	22.2

trimmed by curved scissors (Fig 20-2). In most cases the base of the scrotal skin can be inverted into the surgical wound and the tab of the prosthetic testis is sutured to the bottom of the scrotal compartment with a 3-0 chromic catgut suture. (If this is not possible, a separate small scrotal incision may be required.) The suture should include the dartos muscle and subcutaneous tissues but should not pass through the skin. The prosthesis is then placed distally by everting the scrotal sac back to its usual position. The neck of the upper scrotal tissues above the prosthesis is closed with a 3-0 chromic catgut suture to prevent upward retraction.

When orchiectomy has been done previously, a direct scrotal approach is employed, using one of various types of scrotal incisions. An upper transverse scrotal incision reduces the risk of eroding the prosthetic through the scrotal wound (Fig 20-3). A lateral or midline raphe incision also may be used. Following appropriate insertion and distal fixation of the prosthesis, as described above, the scrotal incision is closed with interrupted 4-0 chromic catgut on the dartos

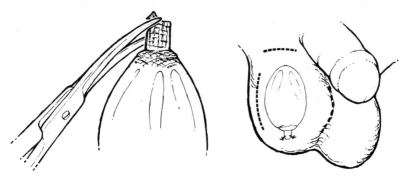

Fig 20-2 (left).—Sharp corners of Silastic tab are trimmed with curved scissors.

Fig 20-3 (right).—Prosthetic testis may be inserted through inguinal wound or at a later procedure through a variety of possible scrotal incisions: upper scrotal, scrotal raphe, or lateral *(dashed lines)*.

layer and 4–0 plain catgut or Dexon subcuticular suture to oppose the skin edges. The scrotal skin wound is then sealed with a collodion dressing.

Two possible major complications observed after testicular prosthetic insertion are rejection and infection. In teenagers, a scrotal support may be used for seven to 10 days postoperatively. Although all children should refrain from vigorous physical exercise for three weeks, complete bedrest, as advocated for adults, is unnecessary.

In instances of anorchism, a bilateral testicular prosthesis should be inserted, followed by a course of exogenous testosterone therapy to complete and maintain male sexual maturation. Such treatment is best initiated at 13 or 14 years of age. Testosterone enanthate (100 mg/ml) is given intramuscularly twice monthly.[26] Complications related to this therapy include advanced bone age and, occasionally, frequent and prolonged erections. If bone age progresses too rapidly, testosterone treatment may be discontinued for a six-month period and resumed at a later time using a lower dose schedule.

REFERENCES

1. Benson C.D., Lofti M.W.: The pouch technique in the surgical correction of cryptorchidism in infants and children. *Surgery* 62:967, 1967.
2. Cywes C.: Undescended testis: Symposium on Long-Term Follow-up in Congenital Anomalies, Pittsburgh Children's Hospital, Pittsburgh, 1979.
3. Gross R.E., Jewett T.C. Jr.: Surgical experiences from 1,222 operations for undescended testes. *J.A.M.A.* 160:634, 1956.
4. Hortling H., Chappelle A., Johansson C.J., et al.: An endocrinologic follow-up study of operated cases of cryptorchidism. *J. Clin. Endocrinol. Metab.* 27:120, 1967.
5. Sudmann E.: The undescended testis: A clinical and histologic study. *Acta Chir. Scand.* 137:815, 1971.
6. Woolley M.M.: Cryptorchidism, in Ravitch M., Welch K., Benson C., et al. (eds.): *Pediatric Surgery*, ed. 3. Chicago, Year Book Medical Publishers, 1979.
7. Levitt S.B., Kogan S.J., Engel R.M., et al.: The impalpable testis: A rational approach to management. *J. Urol.* 120:515, 1978.
8. Fonkalsrud E.W.: The undescended testis, *Curr. Probl. Surg.* 15:1, 1978.
9. Aynsley-Green A., Zachmann M., Illig R., et al.: Congenital bilateral anorchia in childhood: A clinical, endocrine and therapeutic evaluation of 21 cases. *Clin. Endocrinol.* 5:381, 1976.
10. Lee P.A., Hoffman W.H., White J.J., et al.: Serum gonadotropins in cryptorchidism. *Am. J. Dis. Child.* 127:530, 1974.
11. Bramble F.J., Houghton A.L., Eccles S.: Reproductive and endocrine function after surgical treatment of bilateral cryptorchidism. *Lancet* 2:311, 1974.
12. Rivarola M.A., Bergada C., Cullen M.: HCG stimulation test in prepubertal boys with cryptorchidism, bilateral anorchia and in male pseudohermaphroditism. *J. Clin. Endocrinol. Metab.* 31:526, 1970.

13. Levitt S.B., Kogan S.J., Schneider K.M., et al.: Endocrine tests in phenotypic children with bilateral impalpable testes can reliably predict "congenital anorchism." *Urology* 11:11, 1978.
14. Abeyaratne M.R., Aherne W.A., Scott L.S.: The vanishing testes. *Lancet* 2:822, 1969.
15. Jimenez J.F., Lopez-Pacios M.A., Sole-Balcells F.: Anorchia. *Eur. Urol.* 3: 165, 1977.
16. Ehrlich R.M., Dougherty L.J., Tomashefsky P., et al.: Effect of gonadotropin in cryptorchidism. *J. Urol.* 102:793, 1969.
17. Flinn R.A., King L.R.: Experiences with the midline transabdominal approach in orchiopexy. *Surg. Gynecol. Obstet.* 131:285, 1971.
18. Boley S.J., Kleinhaus S.A.: A place for the Cheatle-Henry approach in pediatric surgery. *J. Pediatr. Surg.* 1:394, 1966.
19. Clatworthy H.W. Jr., Hollabaugh R.S., Grosfeld J.L.: The "long-loop vas" orchiopexy for the high undescended testis. *Am. Surg.* 38:69, 1972.
20. Barnhouse D.H.: Prune-belly syndrome. *Br. J. Urol.* 44:356, 1972.
21. Woodard J.R., Parrott T.S.: Orchiopexy in the prune-belly syndrome. *Br. J. Urol.* 50:348, 1978.
22. Scott L.S.: Fertility in cryptorchidism. *Proc. R. Soc. Med.* 55:1047, 1962.
23. Retief P.J.M.: Fertility in undescended testes. *S. Afr. Med. J.* 52:610, 1977.
24. Jewett R.R.: Cryptorchidism: Symposium on Long-Term Follow-up in Congenital Anomalies, Pittsburgh Children's Hospital, Pittsburgh, 1979.
25. Lattimer J.K., Vakili B.F., Smith A.M., et al.: A natural feeling testicular prosthesis. *J. Urol.* 110:81, 1973.
26. Pinch L., Aceto T., Meyer-Bahlburg H.F.: Cryptorchidism. *Urol. Clin. North. Am.* 3:573, 1974.

21 / Results Following Orchiopexy

S. CYWES, M.D.

P.J.M. RETIEF, M.B.

J.H. LOUW, M.CH.

IT IS GENERALLY AGREED that the chief objective in treatment of undescended testes is to prevent progressive degeneration of spermatogenesis. However, there is considerable disagreement regarding what constitutes optimal therapy and at what age it should be provided.

Two basic views regarding optimum age are represented: orchiopexy between three and six years of age, and orchiopexy after age 10. This controversy prompted us to study the long-term anatomical, histologic, and functional results in a series of young men who had undergone orchiopexy for unilateral and bilateral undescended testes before puberty.

We compared these results with those reported by others and then analyzed them with respect to the age at which orchiopexy was performed and with respect to certain hormonal and histologic studies of the testes in boys with undescended testes. On the basis of these findings, we propose a policy of treatment that might improve the ultimate objective of orchiopexy, i.e., fertility.

MATERIAL

During the 16-year period between 1956 and 1971, 769 boys with undescended testes were treated by orchiopexy at our children's hospital (Table 21-1). The operations were performed by various surgeons, but the technique used was basically the same for all and conformed to that recommended by Koop and Minor.[1] Of the boys, 567 had unilateral and 202 had bilateral undescended testes. The average age at which orchiopexy was performed was seven to eight years, although our policy at that time was to recommend operation at four to six years of age.

Of the 769 patients, 492 (64%) have thus far been recalled for exami-

TABLE 21-1.— EXPERIENCE WITH ORCHIOPEXY
RED CROSS WAR MEMORIAL CHILDREN'S HOSPITAL (1956-1971)

| | NO. OF PATIENTS | | | NO. OF TESTES |
TREATMENT	UNILATERAL	BILATERAL	TOTAL	
Patients operated on	567	202	769	971
Patients assessed (64%)				
Orchiopexy	323	132	455	587
Orchiectomy	8	–	8	–
Exploration	29	–	29	–
Total	360	132	492	587

nation and assessment. Among these, 132 (26%) underwent bilateral
and 323 (66%) unilateral orchiopexies. Eight had orchiectomies, and
in 29 other patients exploration failed to detect a missing testis and
they were therefore believed to have agenesis. Thus 587 testes were
available for assessment.

Four hundred and five (69%) of the testes had been truly undescended. Forty-seven percent of the 587 testes were emergent or high
scrotal, 16% were entrant (intracanicular), and 6% were abdominal.
Of the 587 testes, 26% had been ectopic, 24% superficial inguinal,
1.5% perineal (characteristic in pigs), and 0.2% crural. None was pu-
bopenile (characteristic in kangaroos).

RESULTS

Anatomical and Cosmetic Results

All 492 patients were examined and evaluated by one independent
observer—a urologic surgeon,[2] who considered size, consistency, position, and mobility and judged these factors as good, fair, or poor.

Good—testis 75% the size of the opposite testis (or an average of the
two if 75% of normal in bilateral cases), scrotally placed, of firm consistency, and mobile.

Fair—testis 50-75% of average size, scrotally placed but relatively
fixed, with less firm consistency.

Poor—testis small, less than 50% of average size, not located well
down in the scrotum and fixed, or clearly atrophic.

The overall results were good in 352 (60%), fair in 105 (18%), and
poor in 130 (22%). Of the latter testes, 82 (14%) were clearly atrophic.
Although the good and fair results may be combined to give a 78% satisfactory outcome, the fact remains that the 22% poor results must be
regarded as failures of treatment. It should be noted that, in some patients, there was no increased growth spurt at puberty, even though

TABLE 21-2.—COMPARISON OF POSTOPERATIVE ANATOMICAL RESULTS VS. ORIGINAL POSITION OF UNDESCENDED TESTIS*

RATING	EMERGENT	ENTRANT	ABDOMINAL	SUPERFICIAL INGUINAL	PERINEAL	CRURAL
Good	63 (%)	50 (%)	21 (%)	67 (%)	100 (%)	100 (%)
Fair	19	17	6	13	–	–
Poor	18	33	73	20	–	–

*No testis found in 5.

the testis resided well down in the scrotum. Assessment of the anatomical growth of the testis should therefore be guarded until after puberty.

The relationship of the postoperative anatomical location to the original position of the testis is shown in Table 21-2. A clear correlation shows that the higher the testis the poorer the result.

Histologic Results

Histologic biopsies were taken from 41 patients at varying intervals following orchiopexy and these were assessed by one pathologist. Morphological evidence of spermatogenic activity was found in almost all testes that were classified as anatomically good or fair. However, during the course of our investigation, it became apparent that the histologic studies of spermatogenesis often failed to correlate with fertility. Although normal fertility always is associated with normal histologic features, gross deficiencies in seminal fluid also may accompany a near-normal cellular appearance. However, microscopic recognition of spermatogonia at the time of orchiopexy may provide useful information regarding the spermatogenic potential, even at an early age.

The results of the biopsies were good, 17 (41%); fair, 8 (20%); poor, 7 (17%); and atrophic, 9 (22%).

Fertility

Inasmuch as paternity alone is an unreliable indicator, semen was analyzed in appraisal of fertility. Specimens of seminal fluid were classified as good, fair, or poor, classification being based mainly on density of the spermatozoa. Those rated as good had a count of more than 60 million spermatozoa per milliliter; fair, 20 – 60 million/ml; and poor, less than 20 million/ml. For borderline counts the motility and morphologic characteristics of spermatozoa were useful in determining the classification. A small volume of fluid, less than 0.5 ml, tended to be associated with other unfavorable features.

In this study, 29 men with bilateral and 76 with unilateral undescent were sexually mature enough for semen analysis. Their average age was 19 years (range, 15 to 26 years). Semen analyses were performed by one technician; all low counts were repeated and the most favorable of the counts was accepted. Seminal fluid obtained from several normal men who had been proved to be fertile was used as controls. Findings for the 29 men who underwent bilateral orchiopexy are shown in Table 21–3. Surprisingly, a satisfactory anatomical result was obtained in 90% of this small group. Although a satisfactory histologic appearance was present in 12 of 16 (75%) of those on whom biopsies were performed, semen of good quality was obtained in just over 10%. In fact, the semen was of such inferior quality in 66% that these men were most likely sterile.

The results of this small series indicate that 66% of the men will not father children and, at best, 34% will be capable of paternity to varying degrees; only 10% are likely to become fathers. It is interesting to note that 10 patients who experienced good anatomical results had poor semen analyses; two of these were azoospermic. Thus neither anatomical excellence nor normal histologic results are reliable indicators of fertility.

The question of fertility relative to bilateral testicular undescent treated by orchiopexy before puberty has been studied during the past three decades.[3-8] All of the investigators have accepted a semen count exceeding 20 million/ml as evidence of fertility, and on this basis 10 of our 29 patients (34%) who required bilateral orchiopexy can be classified as fertile. This finding compares well with the overall figure of 29% based on semen analysis (Table 21–4).

To assess male fertility, the apparent normality of the testis, epididymis, and vasa must be clinically established. If seminal fluid can be produced, the prostate and seminal vesicles must be functioning; if spermatozoa are seen, the ducts from the testes also are patent. Fertili-

TABLE 21–3.—RESULTS FOLLOWING ORCHIOPEXY
FOR BILATERAL UNDESCENDED TESTIS (29 PATIENTS)

	SEMEN		HISTOLOGY		ANATOMICAL POSITION	
RATING	NO.	%	NO.	%	NO.	%
Good	3	10	8	50	20	69
Fair	7	24	4	25	6	21
Poor	13	45	3	19	2	10
Sterile	6	21	1	6	1°	

°Atrophic.

TABLE 21-4.—FERTILITY IN BILATERAL
CRYPTORCHID PATIENTS TREATED BY
PREPUBERTAL ORCHIOPEXY

AUTHOR	NO. OF PATIENTS	NO. FERTILE	%
McCollum (1935)	22	15	68
Hansen (1949)	25	2	8
Rea (1951)	9	0	0
Maitland (1953)	7	2	29
Hand (1955)	27	15	55
Gross and Jewett (1956)	16	12	75
Brunet et al. (1958)	6	3	50
Bergstrant (1960)	25	14	56
Scott (1962)	12	2	17
Albescu et al. (1971)	11	3	27
Bramble et al. (1974)	21	10	48
Atkinson et al. (1975)	18	8	44
Present study (1976)	29	10	34

ty is assessed chiefly on the basis of quantity and quality of the sper-matozoa. Although theoretically only one healthy spermatozoon is needed to fertilize an ovum, the chance of impregnation is meager unless spermatozoa are present in sufficient numbers.

Earlier investigators set the density of spermatozoa below which the possibility of pregnancy was reduced at 60 million/ml based on the fact that 75% of known fathers had spermatozoa counts over 60 million/ml and 25% had counts ranging from 20 to 60 million/ml.[9] Eventually it was internationally agreed that the standard for paterni-ty should be at least 20 million/ml, coupled with good motility and morphology.[10, 11] Moreover, reliability of the sperm count depends on the method of collection and the technique employed.

Our study, which used the stricter criterion of 60 million spermato-zoa per milliliter, demonstrated that only 10% of men with bilateral undescended testes treated by orchiopexy before puberty were fer-tile. We believe this to be a realistic assessment of good fertility.

When assessing fertility in men with unilateral testicular descent, it should be noted that semen analysis reflects only the overall function-al ability (Table 21-5). In contrast to the men with bilateral unde-scent, only 54% achieved a satisfactory anatomical result, and only 52% of those who had biopsies demonstrated satisfactory histologic results. Fertility in this group was clearly impaired: 35% were as-sessed as having good fertility and 33% reduced fertility, constituting 68% with varying degrees of possible paternity. Among them, 28%

TABLE 21-5.—Results Following Orchiopexy
for Unilateral Undescended Testis (76 Patients)

RATING	SEMEN		HISTOLOGY		ANATOMICAL POSITION	
	NO.	%	NO.	%	NO.	%
Good	27	35	9	36	22	29
Fair	25	33	4	16	19	25
Poor	21	28	4	16	13	46
Sterile	3	4	8	32	22°	–

°Atrophic.

are unlikely to become fathers; 4% are sterile—significantly more than the expected 1% among the general male population.

Serum Gonadotropins

Serum LH and FSH levels were measured in 41 men who had had a unilateral orchiopexy and in 18 who had had bilateral orchiopexies before puberty. At the same time, the testosterone level was measured and a full semen analysis was carried out. The FSH radioimmunoassay was performed by using the FSH radioimmunoassay kit (normal range, 3-16 mIU/ml), and the LH level was measured by a double antibody radioimmunoassay according to the method of Midgley[12] (normal range, 3-15 mIU/ml).

Table 21-6 summarizes the results of sperm count, LH, FSH, and testosterone concentrations in these patients. Figures 21-1 and 21-2 depict the serum FSH values in relation to the semen count after unilateral and bilateral orchiopexy, respectively. Elevated levels were found in 11 of the 41 men subsequent to unilateral and in 11 of the 18 men after bilateral orchiopexy. Of the 11 men who had elevated FSH semen levels in the unilateral group, five had a semen count below 20 million/ml and in the bilateral group, of the 11 with raised FSH levels, 10 had counts below 20 million/ml (Table 21-7).

Thus there was no obvious relationship between sperm count and plasma FSH other than that most elevated levels were associated with oligospermia.

DISCUSSION

The subfertility encountered in our patients after orchiopexy for unilateral undescent is generally consistent with the findings of other investigators (Table 21-8). In the study published by Albescu et al.,[3] patients with palpably small testes were excluded, hence the high fertility rate. A recent study of 17 patients by Gottschalk et al.[13] found

TABLE 21-6.–COMPARISON OF SPERM COUNT WITH LH, FSH, AND TESTOSTERONE VALUES

UNILATERAL UNDESCENDED TESTES

GROUP MIL/ML	NO. OF PATIENTS	SPERM COUNT			LH MIU/ML			FSH MIU/ML			TESTOSTERONE NMOL/L		
		MEAN	SD	RANGE	MEAN	SD	RANGE	MEAN	SD	RANGE	MEAN	SD	RANGE
>60	8	99.2	25.73	64-145	8.1	3.29	3.8-13.1	12.0	4.42	4.8-18.3	21.6	3.39	16.5-25.8
20-60	19	34.0	11.13	20.5-55	11.4	5.12	2.9-20.9	13.1	7.22	4.0-32.5	26.2	6.34	17.9-44.7
<20	12	9.0	5.58	0.1-19	9.7	3.86	3.3-15.8	15.1	4.10	8.9-22.4	23.0	6.24	11.6-32.2
Azoospermia	2	0	0	0	11.5	6.93	6.6-16.4	18.7	5.44	14.8-22.5	23.0	0.21	22.8-23.1

BILATERAL UNDESCENDED TESTES

GROUP MIL/ML	NO. OF PATIENTS	SPERM COUNT			LH MIU/ML			FSH MIU/ML			TESTOSTERONE NMOL/L		
		MEAN	SD	RANGE	MEAN	SD	RANGE	MEAN	SD	RANGE	MEAN	SD	RANGE
>60	0	–	–	–	–		–	–		–	–		–
20-60	2	30	7.07	25-35	12.9	2.55	11.1-14.7	15.2	6.36	10.7-19.7	42.8	18.67	29.6-56.0
<20	11	5.67	5.73	0.15-16	13.1	3.07	8.5-18.7	20.5	5.47	13.4-31.0	26.0	4.95	16.7-32.2
Azoospermia	5	0	0	0	9.7	5.44	3.4-17.9	18.5	13.22	6.9-38.5	22.1	7.93	13.6-34.3

Normal values:
LH – 3-16 mIU/ml
FSH – 3-16 mIU/ml
Testosterone – 10-35 nMol/L

Mil = million; mIU = milli-International Units; nMol = nanomole.

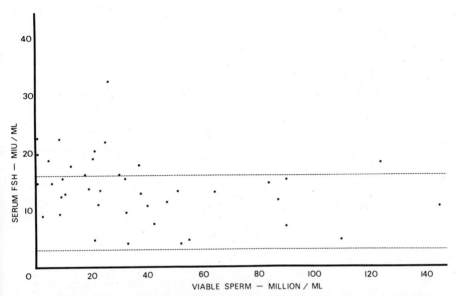

Fig 21–1.—Serum FSH levels in relation to sperm count in men who had undergone unilateral prepubertal orchiopexy. Range of normal values is indicated by the two horizontal *dashed lines.*

infertility in three, restricted fertility in four, and extremely restricted fertility in 10. No patient was deemed to have good fertility. The studies of Mengel et al.[14] in 237 boys with unilaterally undescended testes have provided evidence that there is a significant decrease in spermatogonia content and average tubular diameter in 90% of unilaterally undescended testes. More important, however, is the observation that 15% of the boys had complete loss and 53% a substantial decrease in spermatogonia and failure of tubular development in the contralateral normally descended testis; in other words, in only 32% was normal germinal epithelium observed. We have been able to confirm this in a small number of patients, as have Gottschalk et al.[13]

Figure 21–3, A, shows very poor spermatogenesis of an undescended testis in a 22-year-old man. Figure 21–3, B, illustrates the clearly subnormal histologic features of the contralateral normally descended testis, i.e., inadequate lumen formation and relatively small, rounded tubules with peritubular fibrosis. Although spermatogenesis is present, a specimen of semen from this man was analyzed as follows: volume 1.5 ml; count, 20 million/ml; motility, 30%; and morphologically abnormal sperm, 40%—all of which indicate subfertility. The mecha-

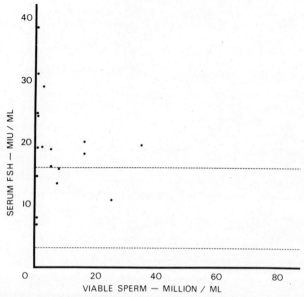

Fig 21–2. — Serum FSH levels in relation to sperm count in men who had undergone bilateral prepubertal orchiopexy. Range of normal values is indicated by the two horizontal *dashed lines*.

nism of the damage to the normal-appearing descended testis is still unknown.

Shirai et al.[15] demonstrated in dogs that when unilateral cryptorchidism is experimentally induced, not only the retained but also the scrotal testis is irreversibly damaged. If, however, the retained testis

TABLE 21–7. — POST-ORCHIOPEXY
COMPARISON OF SPERM COUNTS AND
FSH VALUES

UNILATERAL UNDESCENDED TESTES	
Normal FSH + normospermia	21 (51.2%)
Normal FSH + oligospermia	9 (22.0%)
Raised FSH + normospermia	6 (14.6%)
Raised FSH + oligospermia	5 (12.2%)
Total	41
BILATERAL UNDESCENDED TESTES	
Normal FSH + normospermia	1 (5.6%)
Normal FSH + oligospermia	6 (33.3%)
Raised FSH + normospermia	1 (5.6%)
Raised FSH + oligospermia	10 (55.5%)
Total	18

Oligospermia <20 million/ml.

TABLE 21–8.—Fertility in Unilateral
Cryptorchid Patients Treated by
Prepubertal Orchiopexy

AUTHOR	NO. OF PATIENTS	NO. FERTILE	%
Hansen (1949)	36	15	42
Albescu et al. (1971)	14	13	93
Atkinson et al. (1975)	42	32	76
Lipschultz (1976)	29	21	72
Present study (1976)	76	52	68

is returned to its original place after three months, the lesions of both testes are reversible. These findings have been confirmed by Gottschalk et al.[13]

It has been suggested that the undescended testis produces a substance that impairs the function of the otherwise contralateral normally descended testis. However, Woodhead et al.[16] demonstrated that men with a unilaterally undescended testis previously treated by orchiectomy had the same rate of subnormal sperm density as those who

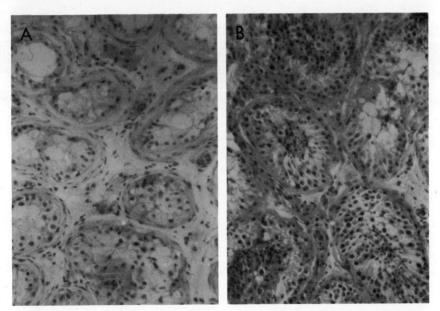

Fig 21–3.—A, histologic appearance of undescended testis from 22-year-old man showing poor spermatogenesis. **B,** histologic appearance of contralateral normally descended testis, which is clearly subnormal, with inadequate lumen formation and small, rounded tubules with peritubular fibrosis.

still retained the unilaterally undescended testis. This makes production of a harmful substance by the undescended testis less likely and probably indicates a primary fault in the descended testis. Various hormonal studies conducted in infertile patients support the latter concept.

Hormonal studies relating to undescended testes are discussed in greater detail elsewhere in this book, but certain aspects are pertinent to the results of orchiopexy. For example, it is now apparent that in the presence of a normal pituitary gland, severe bilateral testicular damage is associated with elevated levels of FSH. De Kretser et al.[17] have shown that a significant correlation exists between serum FSH levels and the mean number of spermatogonia per tubule, and that elevated levels of FSH in plasma of azoospermic patients almost invariably indicate severe testicular destruction. They suggest that the higher FSH levels probably reflect diminished inhibition of FSH secretion by a presumed, but as yet unidentified, product of the seminiferous tubules.

Lipschultz et al.[18] carried out hormone studies on patients who had undergone orchiopexies for unilaterally undescended testes during boyhood (four to 12 years of age). They found that, although the mean sperm density in these men was only one-third that of normal, their serum testosterone level did not differ significantly from that of a control group. However, their FSH levels were significantly higher than those in normal men, and their response to LH-RH was more than double that for normal males. These results led to the conclusion that, in patients with unilaterally undescended testes, both testes must be abnormal.

In contrast, a recent Swiss and German collaborative study by Illig et al.[19] on the effect of intranasal LH-RH on unilaterally and bilaterally undescended testes noted that after four weeks' treatment, complete descent occurred in 38% of 61 testes, an improved position in 28%, and no response in 19%; 15% of the testes were never palpated. The success rate was independent of age and laterality, but was related to the initial testicular position, complete descent occurring in only 11% of impalpable testes compared with 48% of inguinal testes. In controls who were given a placebo, only one of 51 testes descended completely, whereas the position of the testes improved in 15%. The probable explanation of these conflicting findings is that undescended testes represent a spectrum of disorders with a local testicular fault at one extreme and a fault in gonadotropic secretion at the other.

As reported in *Lancet* of June 1978,[20] other workers have obtained similar results with subcutaneous or intramuscular injections of LH-

RH. Fertility has not yet been assessed in these patients. Nevertheless, if we can prevent the need of orchiopexy in a third of our patients by prescribing these hormones, such a regimen can be considered a worthwhile form of treatment.

An important aspect of the study by Mengel et al.[14] demonstrated that, although germinal epithelium of undescended testes was not visibly damaged during the first two years of life, during the third year a significant drop in spermatogonia content and decrease in tubular diameter occurred. These findings have been confirmed by Gottschalk et al.[13] and by the pathologists at our hospital. Figure 21–4, A, shows a normal-appearing testis in a three-year-old boy (autopsy specimen); Figure 21–4, B, shows an undescended testis from a boy of the same age (biopsy specimen). The frequent spermatogonia in the normal testis contrast with the tubular atrophy and infrequent spermatogonia in the undescended testis. These changes exacerbate in extent and frequency during subsequent years.

Figure 21–5 shows the histologic results at 10 years: maturing tubules and spermatogonia in the normal testis, and atrophic tubules with minimal spermatogonia in the undescended testis. Figure 21–6

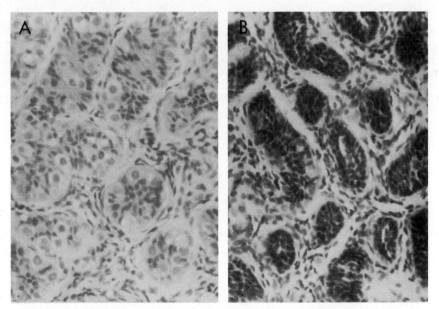

Fig 21–4.—Biopsies of testes at age three. **A,** normal histologic appearance with frequent spermatogonia (autopsy specimen). **B,** biopsy specimen of undescended testis showing tubular atrophy and infrequent spermatogonia.

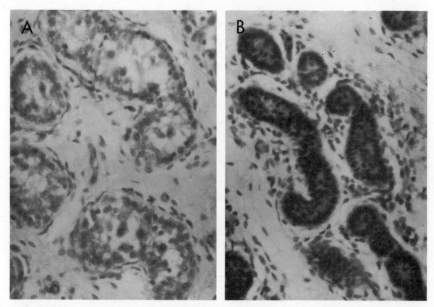

Fig 21–5.—Histologic appearance at 10 years of age: **A,** normal control; **B,** undescended testis. Note maturing tubules and spermatogonia in normal testis and atrophic tubules with scanty spermatogonia in undescended testis.

shows the histologic appearance at age 12½ years. Maturing tubules with spermatocytes are evident in the normal testis, but inactive tubules with surrounding fibrosis appear in the undescended testis.

On the other hand, Kiesewetter et al.[21] demonstrated that the histologic appearance of the testis can improve after orchiopexy. In their study of 29 patients in whom they staged the procedure, they were able to compare the histologic appearance of the same testis before and after orchiopexy; the results showed a moderate to marked improvement in 52% of these testes, slight improvement in 34%, and no change in 14%. In an experimental model Kiesewetter et al.[22] also demonstrated improvement in size and histologic appearance after returning the testis to the scrotum following six months in an undescended position.

Scott[7] noted some impairment of fertility in two thirds of untreated unilateral cryptorchid patients, whereas three quarters of his patients who had undergone orchiopexy before age five were fully fertile. Thus the optimum age for orchiopexy is obviously of great importance. Hecker et al.[23] as well as Mengel et al.,[14] strongly recommend that orchiopexy be performed before the end of the second year of life. In-

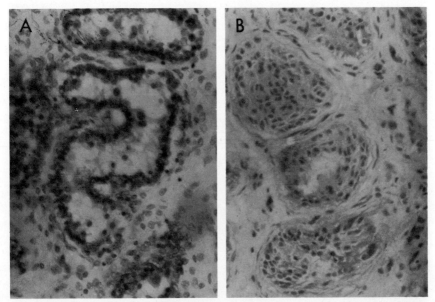

Fig 21–6.—Histologic appearance at 12½ years of age. **A,** normal control showing maturing tubules with spermatocytes (autopsy specimen); **B,** biopsy of undescended testis showing inactive tubules with surrounding fibrosis.

deed, for many years Koop[1] has been doing the operation as soon as possible after the age of six months. Whitaker[24] advised orchiopexy during the first year of life if the undescended testis is ectopic or associated with an obvious hernia.

Ludwig and Potempa[25] in 1975 reported on fertility based on semen analysis relative to the age at orchiopexy. In a group of 71 children who had undergone orchiopexies for unilateral undescent between 1950 and 1960, these authors found that 87.5% (eight patients) of those repaired between ages one and two years were fertile; 57.1% (seven patients) repaired between ages three and four were fertile, as were 38.5% (26 patients) repaired between ages five and eight, 25% (16 patients) repaired between ages nine and 12 years, and only 14.3% (14 patients) repaired after age 13.[25] Therefore they recommend orchiopexy (at the latest) before the end of the second year.

Although it is generally agreed that successful surgical placement of a testis low in the scrotum is preferable in young children, this advantage is offset by the fact that the very flimsy membrane of the hernia sac surrounding an infant's undescended testis makes dissection very difficult and increases the risk of injury to the spermatic cord and testis. However, in experienced hands, and with meticulous operative technique, the favorable anatomical results alone make it worthwhile. If, in addition, significantly improved chances of fertility are achieved, orchiopexy at age two years becomes mandatory. Indeed, this has been the policy at our hospital for the past three years. It has been suggested that treatment with a short course of hormonal therapy be started when the child is between one and two years of age, and if the testis has not completely descended at two years, orchiopexy should then be performed.[20]

CONCLUSIONS

From our survey we conclude that subsequent to orchiopexy for undescended testes performed at seven to eight years, the following may be expected:

1. A satisfactory anatomical outcome in four out of five patients.

2. A satisfactory histologic result in two out of three patients.

3. A possibility of parenthood in one third of those with bilaterally undescended testes and in two thirds of those with unilaterally undescended testis.

Our survey also has impressed upon us the importance of the anatomical result to patients and their parents.

There is now abundant evidence that both testes are abnormal even in unilateral cases and that abnormal morphological changes begin to appear during the second year of life. There also is evidence that these changes often may be prevented by bringing the testis into the scrotum before the age of two to three years. Furthermore, as Martin and Menck[26] pointed out, in testes that have been brought down into the scrotum early, there is less likelihood of late malignancy than in gonads brought down later.

In view of these factors, we now advise orchiopexy at the age of two years. We also believe that if a dysplastic testis cannot be brought down into the scrotum, it should be removed and a prosthesis inserted to prevent an adverse effect on the contralateral testis.

The role of LH-RH therapy for cryptorchidism is currently being assessed (see Chapter 9).

REFERENCES
1. Koop C.E., Minor C.L.: Observations on undescended testes: II. The technique of surgical management. *Arch. Surg.* 75:898, 1957.
2. Retief P.J.M.: Fertility in undescended testes. *S. Afr. Med. J.* 52:610, 1977.
3. Albescu T.Z., Bergada C., Cullen M.: Male fertility in patients treated for cryptorchidism before puberty. *Fertil. Steril.* 22:829, 1971.

4. Bramble F., Houghton A.L., Eccles S., et al.: Reproductive and endocrine function after surgical treatment of bilateral cryptorchidism. *Lancet* 2: 311, 1974.
5. Gross R.E., Jewett T.C. Jr.: Surgical experiences from 1,222 operations for undescended testis. *J.A.M.A.* 160:634, 1956.
6. Jansen T.S.: Fertility in operatively treated and untreated cryptorchidism. *Proc. R. Soc. Med.* 42:645, 1949.
7. Scott L.S.: Fertility in cryptorchidism. *Proc. R. Soc. Med.* 55:1047, 1962.
8. Atkinson P.M.: A follow-up study of surgically treated cryptorchid patients. *J. Pediatr. Surg.* 10:115, 1975.
9. Hotchkiss R.S., Brunner E.K., Grenley P.: Semen analysis of 200 fertile men. *Am. J. Med. Sci.* 196:362, 1938.
10. Freund M.: Standards for the rating of human sperm morphology: A cooperative study. *Int. J. Fertil.* 11:97, 1966.
11. MacLeod J.: The semen examination. *Clin. Obstet. Gynecol.* 8:115, 1965.
12. Midgley A.R.: Radioimmunoassay: A method for human chorionic gonadotropin and human luteinizing hormone. *Endocrinology* 79:10, 1966.
13. Gottschalk E., Friedrich U., Meerbach W., et al.: Clinical and experimental studies of the problem of maldescended testis. *Z. Kinderchir.* 22:51, 1977.
14. Mengel W., Hienz H.A., Sippe W.G., et al.: Studies on cryptorchidism: A comparison of histological findings in germinative epithelium before and after the second year of life. *J. Pediatr. Surg.* 9:445, 1974.
15. Shirai M., Matsushita S., Ichijo S., et al.: Histological changes of the scrotal testis in unilateral cryptorchidism. *J. Exp. Med.* 90:363, 1966.
16. Woodhead D.M., Pohl D.R., Johnson D.E.: Fertility of patients with solitary testes. *J. Urol.* 109:66, 1973.
17. De Kretser D.M., Burger H.G., Hudson B.: The relationship between germinal cells and serum FSH levels in males with infertility. *J. Clin. Endocrinol. Metab.* 38:787, 1974.
18. Lipschultz L.I., Caminos-Torres R., Greenspan C.S., et al.: Testicular function after orchidopexy for unilaterally undescended testis. *N. Engl. J. Med.* 295:15, 1976.
19. Illig R., Kollman F., Borkenstein M., et al.: Treatment of cryptorchidism by intranasal synthetic luteinizing hormone releasing hormone. *Lancet* 2: 518, 1977.
20. Cryptorchidism and gonatrophin therapy, editorial. *Lancet* 1:1344, 1978.
21. Kiesewetter W.B., Schull W.R., Fetterman G.H.: Histological changes in testis following anatomically successful orchidopexy. *J. Pediatr. Surg.* 4: 59, 1969.
22. Kiesewetter W.B., Kalayoglu M., Sachs B.: The effect of abnormal position, scrotal repositioning and human gonadotropic hormone on the developing puppy testis. *J. Pediatr. Surg.* 8:738, 1973.
23. Hecker W.C., Hienz H.A., Mengel W.: Frühbehandlung des Maldescensus Testis. *Dtsch. Med. Wochenschr.* 97:1325, 1972.
24. Whitaker R.H.: Congenital disorders of the testicle, in Blandy J. (ed.): *Urology.* Oxford, Blackwell Scientific Publications, 1976.
25. Ludwig G., Potempa J.: Der optimale Zeitpunkt der Behandlung des Kryptorchismus. *Dtsch. Med. Wochenschr.* 100:680, 1975.
26. Martin D.C., Menck H.R.: The undescended testis: Management after puberty. *J. Urol.* 114:77, 1975.

22 / Indications and Contraindications for Orchiopexy or Orchiectomy

FRANK HINMAN, JR., M.D.

WHEN DEALING WITH the problem of cryptorchidism, the urologist and the pediatric surgeon tend to believe that the hidden testis can most effectively be brought down to a normal state by orchiopexy. However, if the testis will not form spermatozoa to enhance fertility and yet will be more susceptible to malignancy, this achievement may yield only a cosmetic and psychologic "normality."

Indications for orchiopexy occur in two conditions: (1) bilateral cryptorchidism found before puberty, and (2) unilateral cryptorchidism when the testis is palpable.

Contraindications to orchiopexy have become more apparent as we gain experience. Thus the choice of whether to withhold treatment or to perform an orchiectomy involves increasingly important alternatives: in cases of mental retardation with ejaculatory failure, orchiopexy is of little value, since impregnation is undesirable or impossible; the unilateral abdominal testis often is dysgenic and hence will be both hypospermatogenic and prone to malignancy; if adnexal development is incomplete, effective function subsequent to orchiopexy is precluded; and, finally, the unilaterally undescended testis after puberty has lost its spermatogenic potential and requires removal, not orchiopexy.

Doubtful indications range between these relatively clear-cut categories. When the testis is impalpable but well developed and easily brought down, when it is found to be retractile right up to puberty, or when cryptorchidism is bilateral but detected during or after puberty, the decision in favor of operation must be based on evaluation of all factors in each case.

INDICATIONS FOR ORCHIOPEXY

Bilateral Cryptorchidism Before Puberty

Inasmuch as the retained testis loses its spermatogenic potential at puberty, at least one testis should be brought to the scrotum before that time. Laboratory study is required to detect a correctable endocrine deficiency and minimally includes measurement of serum FSH and interstitial cell-stimulating hormone (ICSH) levels. If no major endocrine abnormality is found, these bilateral cases may warrant a short course of HCG therapy (Table 22–1), since descent occurs in 50–75% of boys in some series.[1,2]

When hormonal therapy fails, operation should immediately be considered, inasmuch as increasing abnormality appears after the fifth year (and perhaps even earlier). Operation should be done when the child is in kindergarten: a committee of the Urology Section of the American Academy of Pediatrics studied the psychologic aspects of genital surgery in childhood and concluded that the period between three and six years of age is optimum (Table 22–2).[3] Moreover it is important for the boy to have a nearly normal external configuration by the time he meets his peers in school.

Operation should begin on the side where the testis is most palpable. If the surgeon believes that the status of that testis is satisfactory after fixation, the poorer side can then be dealt with as if it were unilateral cryptorchidism. This allows removal of the testis, when exposed, if it proves to be abnormal. If the less palpable testis were operated on first, this choice would be impossible because technical problems might prevent healthy positioning of the better testis.

TABLE 22–1.—HUMAN CHORIONIC GONADOTROPIN TREATMENT

SOURCE	COURSE	UNITS	INTERVAL	TOTAL
Robinson and Engle[32]	Short	4,000	Daily	12,000
Deming[33]	Long	250	2–3 times a wk	3,000
Hand[34]	Long	4,000	3 times a wk	40,000

TABLE 22–2.—PSYCHOLOGIC
CONSIDERATIONS IN TIMING
PEDIATRIC OPERATIONS

AGE OF CHILD	PSYCHOLOGIC RESPONSE°
0–6 mo	Minimally concerned over brief separation
6–12 mo	Aware of and upset by separation
1–3 yr	Traumatized by separation
3–6 yr	Can be prepared for operation
6 yr and up	Anxious over operations on genitalia (maximally at puberty)

°Separation from parent.

Unilateral Palpable Cryptorchidism Before Puberty

Although it has not been proved (Fig 22–1),[4] fertility may be enhanced by early fixation of the retained testis, especially since a testis palpable "in the canal" may at operation be found retracted laterally into the superficial (Denis-Browne) pouch. Inasmuch as such testes are normal and easily brought down, they probably will function well, with minimal risk of future neoplasia. Those lying within the canal itself can be palpated only when they move down to the external ring; when they are within the canal, the posterior wall of the canal is easily depressed, whereas the overlying external oblique fascia is much stiffer. For these cases, a more extensive dissection is needed, using the principles set down by Prentiss et al.[5] If at operation this technique is inadequate, the testis is probably too abnormal to be functional. In consequence, orchiectomy (supplemented by a Silastic prosthesis for psychologic-cosmetic benefits) is indicated rather than a two-stage operation; resort to division of the spermatic vessels[6]; or a vascular transplantation.[7] The testis must be removed because the risk of subsequent malignancy outweighs the chance of significant fertility enhancement. The parents should be informed of this possibility preoperatively or even during the operation.

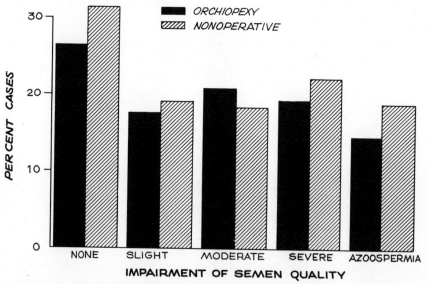

Fig 22–1.—Comparison of semen analysis in treated and untreated cases of unilateral cryptorchidism (353 cases, nine series). (Data from Hinman, *J. Urol.* 122:71, 1979. © 1979, Williams & Wilkins Co., Baltimore. Used with permission.)

In summary, in cases of bilaterally undescended testes before puberty, a definite indication for orchiopexy exists. Although the indication is slightly less strong for the unilateral, partially descended (palpable) testis, orchiopexy is still warranted.

DOUBTFUL INDICATIONS FOR ORCHIOPEXY

Prepubertal Unilateral Well-Developed but Nonpalpable Testis

In a few instances, testes may not have been palpable preoperatively and yet, on exposure in the canal, are of normal size for the child's age (Fig 22–2)[8] and have proper adnexae. Good surgical judgment is required here to balance spermatogenic potential against risk of malignancy.

Parapuberal Retractile Testes

All retractile testes by definition descend when the child is carefully examined under warm water in the bathtub—a good indication for a house call.

Fat boys with small testes, large fat pads, small scrotal sacs, and hyperactive cremasteric reflexes have testes that are at the same temperature as those in the abdomen. As puberty approaches, those few testes remaining at symphyseal level even in a warm bath may require operation.[9] Since the cord is adequate, orchiopexy can be readily accomplished; scrotal size is the only limiting factor.

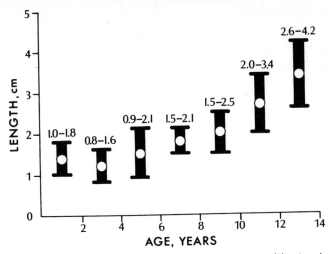

Fig 22–2.—Normal testicular length at various ages, with standard deviations. (Data from Hung et al., *Am. J. Surg.* 138:37, 1979. Used with permission.)

Bilateral Undescended Testes at or After Puberty

There may be some justification for unilateral orchiopexy and contralateral orchiectomy in puberal and postpuberal boys with bilateral nondescent. The chance for fertility is so small and the risk of neoplasm dangerous enough to warrant unilateral orchiectomy rather than bilateral fixation, although most cases are probably best managed without operation. This is especially true if the condition is due to hypopituitarism, since the testes will be neither fertile nor perhaps more prone to neoplasm. Mere placement of prostheses is enough.

The conditions characterized under doubtful indications require good judgment on the part of the surgeon, who should not arbitrarily bring any testis down simply because it is technically possible. Some testes are better left alone or removed.

CONTRAINDICATIONS TO ORCHIOPEXY

Certain classes of cryptorchidism are better managed without orchiopexy, but rather by hormonal therapy or orchiectomy. Besides those who are obviously ill and with poor prognosis, there are three categories of patients who probably should not receive intervention: (1) boys with severe mental incompetency, (2) those with inability to ejaculate effectively, and (3) those with certain major endocrine disorders.

Mental Incompetency

Based on Stanford-Binet (S-B) testing, retardation is customarily divided into four levels. If boys in the severe and profound groups (S-B less than 35) undergo orchiopexy to make fertility possible, a serious social problem is created: the patient and possible offspring will have to be supported, financially and otherwise. In addition, the possibility of fertility would have a restrictive effect on the patient, who would then have to be guarded against opportunities for impregnation. Furthermore, in some instances, heritable disorders could be avoided if orchiopexy were not done.

The deciding factors for or against orchiopexy are often societal rather than medical. The usual contraindications in cases of unilateral cryptorchidism often outweigh the indications. In 50% of children with cerebral damage, testicular development is retarded.[10, 11] Patients with bilateral cryptorchidism, inevitably sterile without surgery, force a decision, not on the surgeon, but on the parents, social workers, and society as a whole.

Ejaculatory Failure

This may be so complete that impregnation is impossible and may occur both in severe neurologic disorders and in the prune belly (triad) syndrome. Consequently, orchiopexy to improve spermatogenesis is futile.

Neurogenic bladder. — This may be accompanied by failure to ejaculate. Boys having myelomeningocele associated with autonomous neurogenic bladder may be expected to have deficient ejaculation and thus, because impregnation would be impossible, orchiopexy is not indicated. Electro-ejaculation[12] may enable the collection of enough semen from patients with high lesions to allow cap insemination, but not from those having lesions at the cauda equina level. Consequently the decision to operate will have to be made after evaluating the sympathetic and parasympathetic deficits of each patient.

Regarding testicular function, no data are available on patients with myelomeningocele, but after traumatic spinal injury, lower sperm counts are common, especially with low lesions.[11]

Triad (prune belly) Syndrome

This syndrome is always associated with some deficiency in ejaculation. Early as well as more recent descriptions of the syndrome (deficient abdominal musculature, urinary tract abnormalities and cryptorchidism) note prostatic tubules in only about one sixth of cases.[13, 14] Severity of the syndrome varies considerably; it may be that mild cases have better prostatic development. However, the difficulties in treating infertility in adult males who have defective vesicular or prostatic fluid but who are otherwise sexually normal suggest that the scanty secretions of the triad syndrome would rarely permit impregnation. Moreover, because the musculature of the posterior urethra is abnormal, leaving a wide pouch in the bottom of which lie the ejaculatory ducts, effective delivery of the fluid is unlikely. What is produced is a pool of semen rather than antegrade propulsion. Adequate ejaculates have not been reported in these patients, although some have occasional emissions.

Malignancies probably occur infrequently, since the testes of the prune belly syndrome are cryptorchid because of failure of the mechanism for descent rather than because of intrinsic testicular abnormalities, as in intra-abdominal testes.

Thus operation is probably not warranted based on hope of fertility or risk of malignancy.

Endocrine Abnormalities

Endocrine anomalies resulting from developmental deficiencies accompanying cryptorchidism may be incompatible with fertility. Chromosomal disturbances, especially Klinefelter's syndrome (with XXY, XXXY, and YY karyotypes) usually cause azoospermia,[15] although fertility is present in some XXY-XY mosaics.[16, 17] Male Turner's syndrome also is accompanied by defective spermatogenesis (and has less hazard of malignancy than does testicular feminization). The Sertoli cell-only syndrome is characterized by germinal cell aplasia. Finally, some male pseudohermaphrodites with inborn errors of testosterone biosynthesis and with certain variants of gonadal dysgenesis appearing as dysgenic male pseudohermaphrodites will be sterile despite orchiopexy. The choice should then be between withholding treatment or performing an orchiectomy.

INDICATIONS FOR HCG OR ORCHIECTOMY

Hormonal Therapy

Although HCG is theoretically harmful,[18] it is probably not so in practice. Its use before operation in bilateral cases has been mentioned.[7] Boys with a single palpable retained testis that is not in the Denis-Browne pouch may respond to hormonal therapy, making operation unnecessary. In any event, a trial of HCG will enable the family and the pediatrician to decide whether operation is or is not necessary. For abdominal testes and those secured lateral to the canal, hormonal therapy is ineffective as well as painful and expensive.

Interest in this form of treatment has varied with the years. The recent report on HCG therapy by Attanasio et al.[1] records better results than those generally achieved in the past (Fig 22–3), i.e., a 62% initial success rate in unilateral cases that fell to 35% after six months. However, these results do not agree with those usually obtained; for instance, older reports on unilateral cases found lower overall responses and poorer results.[19-21]

Luteinizing hormone-release factor has similar therapeutic effects.[20, 21] Illig et al.,[21] using synthetic LH-RF as a nasal spray, obtained descent in 38% of all of 61 cases, but in only 11% if the testes were not previously palpable.

Responses for age at the time of therapy are important, because all treatment should be completed before the child begins school. Much better responses were found in older children, accompanied (perhaps even caused) by a testosterone response twice that of the younger children.[1] But it was also found that success was half as great in boys over age six.[19] In all such studies, some of the testes were retractile and capable of spontaneous descent.[9]

Orchiectomy

The surgeon finds it difficult to advise or carry out orchiectomy for cryptorchidism. Because parents want their son to be normal, they find it difficult to understand why the testis can never become func-

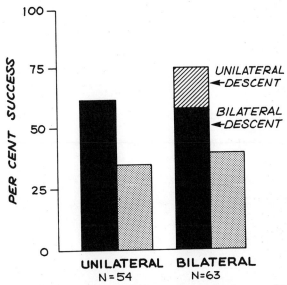

Fig 22–3. – Effect of HCG on cryptorchidism. (Data from Attanasio et al., *J. Endocrinol.* 63:50, 1974.)

tional even though placed in the scrotum. Moreover, the surgeon himself tends to respond to the challenge, devising ingenious techniques. However, if the objectives of improved fertility, cosmetic benefit, and reduction of malignant potential are adhered to, orchiectomy may sometimes be the correct choice.

Removal of the undescended testis is frequently warranted in three conditions: (1) the unilateral abdominal (nonpalpable) testis, (2) the testis failing urogenital union, and (3) the symptomatic unilateral cryptorchid testis after puberty.

Unilateral Abdominal Testis

This condition has undergone review recently regarding the relationship of these testes to fertility, the risk of malignancy, and the psychologic need to be considered.[4] Fertility is probably not enhanced by orchiopexy. The retained testis is frequently dysgenic to a degree roughly proportional to its height intra-abdominally (Fig 22–4).[22] Some available data do not demonstrate improved fertility after orchiopexy for cases of unilateral inguinal cryptorchidism, so that the more abnormal abdominal testis is even less likely to become fertile.

Risk of malignancy is appreciably higher in abdominal testes than in palpable testes (3.3. times) or the normally descended testes of the

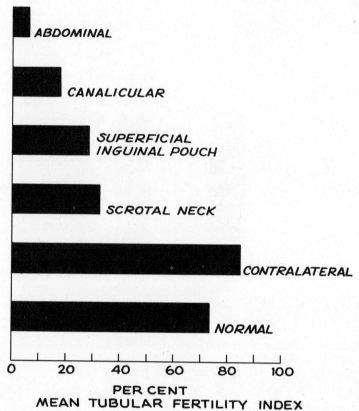

Fig 22–4.–Position and mean tubular fertility index. (Data from Scorer et al., *Campbell's Urology,* vol. 2 [Philadelphia: W. B. Saunders Co., 1979].)

general male population (115 times) (Fig 22–5).[23, 24] Since the unilateral abdominal testis tends to be basically abnormal, the chance that in situ carcinoma will be detected by biopsy at the time of orchiopexy (especially in older boys) is not remote[25, 26] and is a further reason for orchiectomy.[27]

A recent study suggests that orchiopexy does not reduce the incidence of malignancy[28] because the stage at time of diagnosis is similar in the corrected and uncorrected cases (Fig 22–6). Subsequent metastases in patients with stage I and II tumors occur with equal frequency after orchiopexy or spontaneous descent, or in the retained testis. Five-year survival rates of corrected vs. uncorrected cryptorchidism are identical. Moreover, the incidence of metastasis is the same whether the testis is located in the scrotum, groin, or abdomen. In evaluating the possible benefit from orchiopexy, the heightened risk

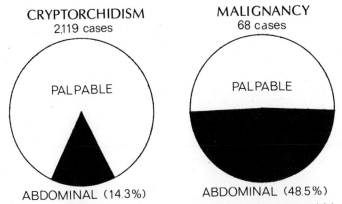

Fig 22–5.—Proportion of abdominal testes among cryptorchid patients and cryptorchid tumors. (Data from Campbell, *Arch. Surg.* 44:353, 1942.)

of inguinal node metastasis must be balanced against the advantage of early detection when the testis is in the scrotum.[29] In the series described by Batata et al.,[28] such metastases occurred in 10% of scrotal and 8% of inguinal testes. The data present a strong argument for operative excision of abdominal testes, since the stage of malignancy at the time of diagnosis appears to be rather high in these cases. In only 50% was malignancy confined to the testis, whereas 14% had distant metastases at that time. Distant metastases appeared later in half of these cases. From these data, it is reasonable to conclude that the abdominal testis, which is doubtfully fertile anyway, presents too high a risk of malignancy to warrant treatment other than removal.

Psychologic benefits can be achieved by use of gel-filled Silastic prostheses; these will be accepted if the parents and the patient are prepared in advance of operation.

Abnormal Adnexae

These defects contraindicate the use of orchiopexy. As many as a quarter of abdominal testes have severe defects of urogenital union, either agenesis of the epididymis or loss of continuity of the vas.[30] Careful examination of these structures at operation may reveal such abnormalities and encourage orchiectomy.

Postpuberal Unilateral Cryptorchidism

This condition requires removal of the testis. The retained testis has lost functional germinal epithelium after puberty, so that improved appearance is all that is gained by orchiopexy. The risk of malignancy overbalances the psychologic benefit of a scrotal testis. Whether orchiectomy is needed for all such testes retained after puberty is based

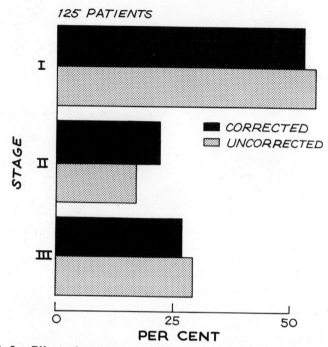

Fig 22–6.—Effect of correction on stage of malignancy. (Data from Batata et al., *Am. J. Roentgenol.* 126:302, 1976.)

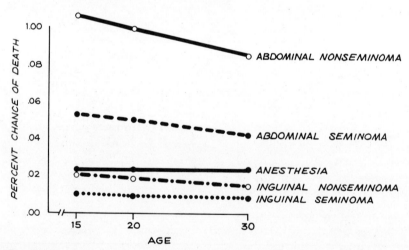

Fig 22–7.—Risk of death from malignancy and operation, assuming cure rates of 95% for seminoma and 85% for nonseminoma. (Data partly from Martin, *J. Urol.* 114:77, 1975.)

on balancing the risk of operation against the danger of future tumor[31] (Fig 22 – 7). Considering the better cure rates now obtained with combined surgery and radiation, a reasonable conclusion is that the nonpalpable testis with its higher chance for malignant change should be removed, whereas the inguinal testis may remain unless it is symptomatic.

SUMMARY

There are various disorders in young males for which concomitant cryptorchidism needs no treatment, or which require treatment by methods other than orchiopexy. Usually, as when fertility is undesirable (severe mental retardation) or impossible (inability to ejaculate because of neurologic abnormalities), no treatment of the undescended testis is required. For unilateral cases in which the testis is either congenitally or chronologically inadequate, removal is preferable to orchiopexy.

REFERENCES
1. Attanasio A., Jendricke K., Bierich J.R., et al.: Clinical and hormonal effect of human chorionic gonadotrophin in prepubertal cryptorchid boys. *J. Endocrinol.* 63:50, 1974.
2. Czaplicki M., Babloc L., Janczewski Z.: Fertility after treatment of bilateral cryptorchidism. *Int. Urol. Nephrol.* 6:259, 1974.
3. A Report by the Action Committee on Surgery of the Genitalia of Male Children: The timing of elective surgery on the genitalia of male children with particular reference to undescended testes and hypospadias. Section of Urology, American Academy of Pediatrics, with the cooperation of the Section on Child Development, American Academy of Pediatrics, 1974.
4. Hinman F. Jr.: Unilateral abdominal cryptorchidism. *J. Urol.* 122:71, 1979.
5. Prentiss R.J., Weickgenant C.J., Moses J.J., et al.: Surgical repair of undescended testicle. *Calif. Med.* 96:401, 1962.
6. Fowler R., Stephens F.D.: The role of testicular vascular anatomy in the salvage of high undescended testes, in Webster R. (ed.): *Congenital Malformations of the Rectum, Anus, and Genito-Urinary Tracts.* London, E & S Livingstone, 1963.
7. Romas N.A., Janecka I., Krisoloff M.: Role of microsurgery in orchiopexy. *Urology* 12:670, 1978.
8. Hung W., August G.P., Glasgow A.M.: *Pediatric Endocrinology.* New York, Medical Examination Publishing Co., 1978.
9. Puri P., Nixon H.H.: Bilateral retractile testes: Subsequent effects on fertility. *J. Pediatr. Surg.* 12:563, 1977.
10. Staedtler F., Hartmann R.: Prepuberal testicular growth in normal boys and those with brain damage. *Dtsch. Med. Wochenschr.* 97:104, 1972.
11. Horne H.W., Paull D.P., Munro D.: Fertility studies in the human male with traumatic injuries of the spinal cord and cauda equina. *N. Engl. J. Med.* 230:959, 1948.

12. François N., Maury M., Jouannet D., et al.: Electro-ejaculation of a complete paraplegic followed by pregnancy. *Paraplegia* 16:248, 1978.
13. Nunn I.N., Stephens F.D.: The triad syndrome: A composite anomaly of the abdominal wall. *J. Urol.* 86:782, 1961.
14. DeKlerk D.P., Scott W.: Prostatic maldevelopment in prune belly syndrome: Defect in prostatic stromal-epithelial interaction. *J. Urol.* 120:341, 1978.
15. Paulsen C.A.: The testis, in Williams R. H. (ed.): *Textbook of Endocrinology.* Philadelphia, W. B. Saunders Co., 1974.
16. Warburg E.: A fertile patient with Klinefelter's syndrome. *Acta Endocrinol. (Copenh.)* 43:12, 1963.
17. Court Brown W.M., Mantle D.J., Buckton K.E., et al.: Fertility in an XY-XXY male married to a translocation heterozygote. *J. Med. Genet.* 1:35, 1964.
18. Heine J.P., Novick H.P., Hinman F. Jr.: Effects of premature puberty on cryptorchid testes in rats. *Surg. Forum* 14:552, 1973.
19. Ehrlich R.M., Dougherty L.J., Tomashefsky P., et al.: Effect of gonadotropin in cryptorchidism. *J. Urol.* 102:793, 1969.
20. Bartsch G., Frick J.: Therapeutic effects of luteinizing hormone releasing hormone (LH-RH) in cryptorchidism. *Andrologia* 6:197, 1974.
21. Illig R., Kollmann F., Borkenstein M., et al.: Treatment of cryptorchidism by intranasal synthetic luteinizing-hormone releasing hormone: Result of a collaborative double blind study. *Lancet* 2:518, 1977.
22. Scorer C.G., Farrington G.H.: Congenital anomalies of the testes: Cryptorchidism, testicular torsion, and inguinal hernia and hydrocele, in Harrison J.H., Gittes R.F., Perlmutter A.D., et al. (eds.): *Campbell's Urology*, vol. 2. Philadelphia, W.B. Saunders Co., 1979.
23. Linke C. A., Kiefer J.H.: Occurrence of testis tumor in undescended testis. *J. Urol.* 82:347, 1959.
24. Campbell H.E.: Incidence of malignant growth of the undescended testicle: A critical and statistical study. *Arch. Surg.* 44:353, 1942.
25. Skakkebaek N.E.: Possible carcinoma in-situ of the testis. *Lancet* 2:516, 1972.
26. Waxman M.: Malignant germ cell tumor in situ in a cryptorchid testis. *Cancer* 38:1452, 1976.
27. Leadbetter G.W.: Incipient germ cell tumor and cryptorchid testis. *Society for Pediatric Urology Newsletter*, May 2, 1979.
28. Batata M.A., Whitmore W.F. Jr., Hilaris B.S., et al.: Cancer of the undescended or maldescended testis. *Am. J. Roentgenol.* 126:302, 1976.
29. Hinman F. Jr., quoted by Charney C.W., Wolgin W. (eds.): in *Cryptorchidism.* New York, Springer-Verlag, 1957.
30. Marshall F.F., Shermeta D.W.: Epididymal abnormalities associated with undescended testis. *J. Urol.* 121:341, 1979.
31. Martin D.C., Menck H.R.: Undescended testis: Management after puberty. *J. Urol.* 114:77, 1975.
32. Robinson J.N., Engle E.T.: Some observations on the cryptorchid testis. *J. Urol.* 71:726, 1954.
33. Deming C.L.: Indications for hormonal treatment of cryptorchidism. *J. Urol.* 77:467, 1957.
34. Hand J.R.: Treatment of undescended testis and its complications. *J.A.M.A.* 164:1185, 1957.

23 / Orchiopexy Using Microvascular Anastomoses

DONALD C. MARTIN, M.D.

IN A SMALL BUT SIGNIFICANT percentage of patients with bilateral undescended testes, the internal spermatic artery and vein are not long enough to permit operative placement of the testes into the scrotum. In such cases the testes are frequently located high in the inguinal region or reside intraperitoneally. Patients with the prune belly syndrome characteristically have intra-abdominal testes with short internal spermatic vessels.

Intra-abdominal testes can be placed into the scrotum only by dividing the internal spermatic artery and vein. The testis and its appendages are then dependent on collateral circulation, primarily via the vessels of the vas deferens. Mixter[1] reported unsatisfactory results with this procedure in 1924, and Wangensteen[2] condemned the operation on the basis of experimental work in the dog. However, Fowler and Stephens[3] studied the blood supply of the human testis with injection and angiographic methods and clearly demonstrated the collateral blood supply and vascular pathways of the testis.

Successful orchiopexy with high division of the internal spermatic vessels has been reported by Fowler and Stephens,[3] Clatworthy et al.,[4] and Brendler and Wulfsohn.[5] Measurement of success was based chiefly on the postoperative size of the testis. There has been no published documentation of the subsequent reproductive function of the testis following this operative procedure. Fowler and Stephens[3] took postoperative biopsies of four patients and identified normal-appearing seminiferous tubules. Each of these authors has noted testicular atrophy in some patients,[3, 5] and Fowler and Stephens[3] found atrophy in four of 12 patients. Clatworthy et al.[4] reported 24 good results in 32 operations when the operative procedure carefully preserved the collateral circulation via the vas deferens. There were only six good results in 11 operations when dissection of the cord structure was performed during orchiopexy and before dividing the spermatic vessels.[4] Brendler and Wulfsohn[5] obtained satisfactory results in five patients.

Fowler and Stephens[3] recommended assessing the adequacy of the collateral circulation by incising the tunica albuginea testis while the internal spermatic vessels are temporarily occluded. Adequate collateral circulation was presumed if bleeding continued. Clearly this is a subjective assessment of blood flow, no doubt variable in individual patients.

Microvascular anastomosis for a wide range of clinical conditions now provides a reliable means of maintaining arterial supply and venous drainage during orchiopexy. Digital replantation; use of skin flaps; and complex grafts of skin, subcutaneous tissues, and bone segments have become routine procedures in plastic and reconstructive surgical centers.

Silber and Kelly[6] reported the first effective orchiopexy using microvascular anastomosis to insure a good vascular supply. Silber[7] has since performed an isograft from one identical twin donor to a brother recipient. In this operation, reanastomosis of the vessels and the vas deferens was successful; postoperatively spermatozoa were found in the ejaculate. Romas et al.[8] have published five cases, and Martin and Salibian[9] two, of microvascular anastomosis to place high undescended testes into the scrotum.

The precise role of testicular transplantation in our surgical practice is still to be established. Most cases in the literature have involved bilateral undescended testes, in which the effectiveness of orchiopexy is essential to the possibility of reproductive function. We do not yet know whether the procedure is justified in patients with a normally descended contralateral testis. The major indication would be positive evidence of impaired fertility in men with unilateral undescended testis, which is likely in view of the reported histologic abnormalities in the descended testis among children with unilateral undescended testes. However, the frequency of infertility in this group of men has not been established, inasmuch as current data are inadequate or incomplete.

Hinman[10] has pointed out the numerous contraindications to orchiopexy in selected patients or groups with multiple severe abnormalities. Clearly, there are circumstances in which such time-consuming, elaborate, and costly surgical procedures are unwarranted, and indeed contraindicated. Nonetheless, in carefully selected patients, the application of microvascular surgery is a means of insuring viability of the testis following orchiopexy for high undescended testes.

EQUIPMENT

The equipment for performing an orchiopexy with microsurgery is similar to that used for other microvascular operations. Apart from an expensive operating microscope, the surgeon's instruments comprise only jeweler's forceps, microscissors, and microvascular clamps. The skills required for the procedure are considerable, achieved only after many hours of practice under the microscope in a suitable laboratory. Ideally the surgery should be a collaborative effort with a urologist or pediatric surgeon working alongside a skilled and experienced microsurgeon.

OPERATIVE PROCEDURE

The undescended testis is exposed through a large inguinal incision. We prefer an incision extending above the inguinal ligament to permit access to the retroperitoneum. Because high undescended testes tend to be intraperitoneal, a combined intra-abdominal and extraperitoneal dissection is necessary.

The internal spermatic vessels are mobilized high up into the retroperitoneum, near their communications with the vena cava (or renal vein) and aorta. The spermatic artery may be 1 mm in diameter or less. Use of optical loupes with ×2.8–6 magnification is important during this phase of the operation. The vessels may be identified and marked with fine nylon sutures prior to division. Collateral blood supply to the testis via the vessels accompanying the vas deferens must be carefully preserved, since they also nourish the vas and testicular appendages.

The deep inferior epigastric artery and vein are suitably located and large enough for use in microvascular anastomosis. These vessels are appreciably larger than the corresponding spermatic vessels to which they will be anastomosed. The epigastric vessels are ligated under the rectus muscle to insure sufficient mobility and length for the anastomosis to the spermatic vessels.

Salibian[11] has developed a block of Silastic material to stabilize the microvascular clamp (Fig 23–1).[3] Interrupted sutures of 10–0 and 11–0 monofilament nylon are used for these small vascular anastomoses. Magnification of at least ×25 is required to anastomose vessels in the range of 1-mm diameter (Fig 23–2). Patency and hemostasis are confirmed under the microscope by occluding the vessel distally and observing patency and blood flow. We have administered heparin to approximate one-half the full heparinizing dose, based on patient size, before releasing the vascular clamps. We used only one dose of hepa-

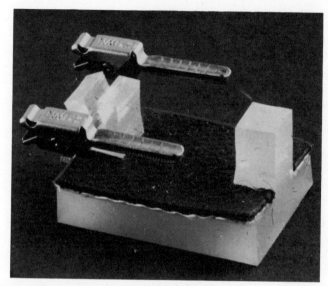

Fig 23–1.—Microvascular clamps supported on Silastic block. This sterilizable supporting block was fashioned by Dr. Arthur Salibian to facilitate microvascular anastomosis in inguinal region.

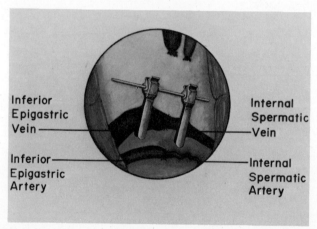

Fig 23–2.—Technique for anastomosis of internal spermatic and inferior epigastric arteries and veins. Epigastric vessels are considerably larger than spermatics.

rin during the operation, followed by low molecular weight dextran, 500 ml during 24 hours, for three days postoperatively to reduce platelet adhesiveness. Division of the internal spermatic vessels high in the retroperitoneum and reanastomosis to the deep inferior epigastric vessels allow adequate length for the surgeon to position the testis in the dependent portion of the scrotum.

Perfusion of the testis is unnecessary and would be extremely difficult owing to the small size of the spermatic artery. However, surface cooling would assist in protecting the testis during the ischemic interval. Cooling to room temperature is adequate for the one or two hours of ischemia needed to complete the vascular anastomoses.

The internal spermatic vein, which is much larger than the artery, is anastomosed first. Not infrequently there will be more than one internal spermatic vein. One large vein should provide adequate venous outflow but if there are two or more small veins, two venous anastomoses might be constructed instead.

Reanastomosis of the artery is the most demanding part of the procedure. The microvascular clamp should stabilize the ends to be anastomosed. The clamp is turned 180 degrees to anastomose the back of the vessel. The anatomical position of the anastomoses is shown in Figure 23–3. Closure of the abdominal wall is performed carefully to avoid angulation or compression of the anastomoses and the internal spermatic vessels.

In the immediate postoperative period, the patency of the vessels may be monitored with a Doppler probe. Radionuclide flow studies also may be used to determine vascularity of the testis, although this procedure does not delineate the pathway through which the blood reaches the testis.

The patency of the microvascular anastomosis was confirmed in one patient by means of selective arteriography (Fig 23–4). Surgical hemoclips were placed in adjacent tissues to identify the site of the vascular anastomoses. The character of the internal spermatic artery is tortuous and distinct from other vessels in the region.

We have performed unilateral orchiopexy using microvascular anastomoses in each of two patients with bilateral intra-abdominal undescended testes. Orchiopexy involving division of the internal spermatic vessels without reanastomosis, while preserving the vessels accompanying the vas, was performed on the contralateral side. The two patients so treated were 10 and 15 years of age, respectively; although both should have received treatment at a younger age, they had not reported for surgery at the appropriate time. We have followed their

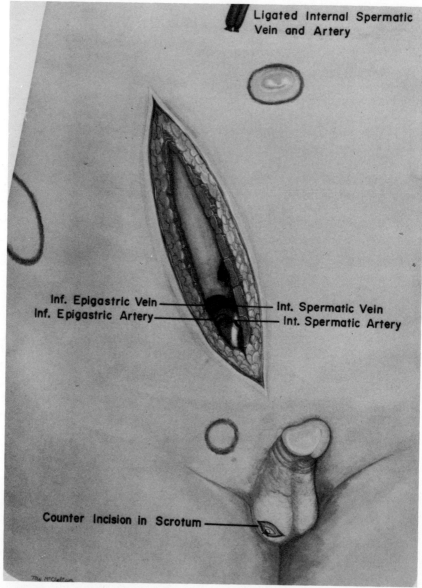

Fig 23–3.—Anatomical relationships during orchiopexy using microvascular anastomosis. Spermatic vessels are ligated near their origin from aorta and vena cava.

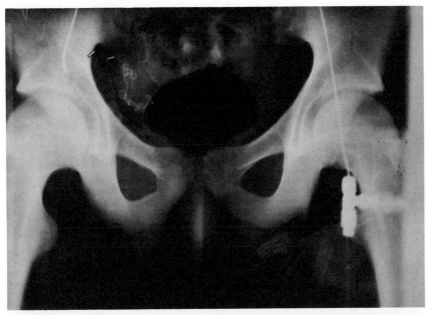

Fig 23–4.—Selective arteriography of deep inferior epigastric artery reveals patency of microvascular anastomosis three months postorchiopexy. Hemoclips mark site of anastomosis. Internal spermatic artery is tortuous. Late x-ray exposures in this study also revealed patency of venous anastomosis. Gonad is present in midscrotum and is of normal size for 15-year-old boy.

progress for two years and found that testicular size is symmetric and appears normal.

During the next few years, testicular biopsies are planned for these patients to assess the status of the microvascular anastomoses. Long-term studies of this type, together with assessment of sperm production, are essential to determine the role of microsurgical reconstruction in treatment of undescended testes.

REFERENCES

1. Mixter C.G.: Undescended testicle: Operative treatment and end results. *Surg. Gynecol. Obstet.* 39:275, 1924.
2. Wangensteen O.H.: Undescended testis: Experimental and clinical study. *Arch. Surg.* 14:663, 1927.
3. Fowler R., Stephens F.D.: The role of testicular vascular anatomy in the salvage of high undescended testes. *Aust. N.Z. J. Surg.* 29:92, 1959.
4. Clatworthy H.W. Jr., Hollabaugh R.S., Grosfeld J.L.: The "long loop vas" orchiopexy for the high undescended testis. *Am. Surg.* 38:69, 1972.

5. Brendler H., Wulfsohn M.A.: Surgical treatment of the high undescended testis. *Surg. Gynecol. Obstet.* 124:605, 1967.
6. Silber S.J., Kelly J.: Successful autotransplantation of an intra-abdominal testis to the scrotum by microvascular technique. *J. Urol.* 115:452, 1976.
7. Silber S.J.: Transplantation of a human testis for anorchia. *Fertil. Steril.* 30:181, 1978.
8. Romas N.A., Janecka I., Krisiloff M.: Role of microsurgery in orchiopexy. *Urology* 12:670, 1978.
9. Martin D.C., Salibian A.: Orchiopexy utilizing microvascular surgical technique. *J. Urol.* In press.
10. Hinman F. Jr.: Unilateral abdominal cryptorchidism. *J. Urol.* 122:71, 1979.
11. Salibian A.: Personal communication.

24 / Summary

ERIC W. FONKALSRUD, M.D.

CRYPTORCHIDISM is one of the most common malformations occurring in males, and much information regarding the embryogenesis and pathophysiologic features of the condition has become available during the past decade. The importance of distinguishing inguinal, abdominal, and ectopic from retractile testes is emphasized by most authors inasmuch as only the latter condition requires no treatment. In general, the higher the location of the testis, the more pronounced are the dysplastic changes and the greater the risk of infertility as well as subsequent malignant transformation.

The hormonal influences effecting testicular descent and the determination of tissue receptor sites are gradually being elucidated so that the optimal initial treatment for most patients is considered by many physicians to be nonoperative. Although HCG may cause descent in about 20% of cryptorchid testes, the initial results with LH-RH are even more encouraging, indicating that this hormone may produce descent in as high as 50% of patients. After a short course of hormone therapy, orchiopexy should be performed on boys who do not obtain complete descent.

The optimal time for initiating treatment for undescent is one to two years of age, since there are valid data indicating that the cryptorchid gonad undergoes progressively severer retardation of normal maturation beyond that age. Although some authors support the view that unilaterally undescended testes that have not been placed in the scrotum by the age of 10 should be removed, most would defer orchiectomy until age 12 to 15, and then only if the gonad is hypoplastic or shows considerable retardation of tubular maturation. There is concern that the unilaterally descended testis is abnormal in about 50% of cases and that fertility is low when dependent on this single gonad.

In patients with bilateral dystopia who do not achieve descent after a course of hormone therapy, orchiopexy is recommended, unless there is a specific contraindication such as severe retardation or CNS disease. Although the standard retroperitoneal dissection through an inguinal incision usually provides good exposure for repair of cryptorchid testes, long-loop vas orchiopexy and transabdominal repair are particularly helpful for high gonads. Clinical experience with autotransplantation and microvascular anastomoses is limited; however, initial reports of success with this technique are encouraging. When both testes are dysplastic, most authors would favor bilateral orchiectomy, insertion of scrotal prostheses, and testosterone replacement. Laparotomy may be necessary to locate high intra-abdominal testes.

The results following placement of the testes into the scrotum either by hormone therapy or orchiopexy depend on the age at which descent occurs, the severity of the dysplastic changes at the time of descent, and the absence of surgical trauma to the gonad and spermatic cord. Sperm counts, tubular fertility index, and spermatogonia appearance on biopsy are more reliable indices of fertility than is successful paternity. Fertility can be anticipated in over 80% of patients with unilateral dystopia in whom descent is produced before three years of age, but the figure decreases rapidly as the age of descent rises. Fertility subsequent to placement of bilateral undescended testes into the scrotum before the age of three years ranges from 40% to 70%.

Malignant degeneration in dystopic testes ranges from 20 to more than 200 times the incidence in normal testes and is highest in intra-abdominal and dysplastic gonads. There is suggestive evidence that early placement of the testis into the scrotum may prevent tubular dysplasia and reduce the incidence of tumor. Only rare cases of tumor have occurred in gonads placed into the scrotum before four years of age. Since high intra-abdominal testes are extremely susceptible to malignant degeneration, particular attention should be directed to locating and removing such gonads if they cannot be placed into the scrotum.

Index